Facilitating Wellness

Inside the Miracle of Hypnosis

Julie Griffin

Illustrated by John Michael Doherty

Author's Photographs by David Hamacher

Cover Design by Bruce Blanchette

 TWT Publishing

Facilitating Wellness

Published by: **TWT Publishing**
Post Office Box 2038
North Chelmsford, MA 01863

A note from the publisher. This book is not meant to serve as a reference guide as to how to treat specific symptoms or cases. All the therapies were designed to meet the specific needs of the individual client.

Publishers Cataloging in Publication

Griffin, Julie.
    Facilitating wellness / Julie Griffin
    p. cm.
    ISBN: 1-57691-001-6.

1. Hypnotism--Therapeutic uses--Case studies.   I. Title.

RC495.G75 1996   615.8512
                        96-60030

for my sister
Abby

About the Author

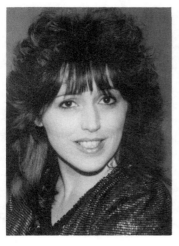

Julie Griffin, C.Ht.**, is a graduate of the American Institute of Hypnotherapy and is a certified instructor of clinical hypnosis. Since 1992 she has conducted over 450 group hypnosis seminars in thirteen states while maintaining a private hypnotherapy practice.

Julie is an active member of The American Board of Hypnotherapy, The International Association of Counselors and Therapists, and The National Guild of Hypnotists.

In 1994, she founded the Hypnotherapy Training Company in Boston, Massachusetts where she directs both basic and advanced hypnotherapy training programs, and was nominated for induction into the International Hypnosis Hall of Fame.

Julie is the author of *Recipes for Wellness*, an inspiring collection of hypnotherapy scripts on a wide variety of topics, as well as *Facilitating Wellness*. Her upcoming books, *Recipes for Living, Recipes for Weight Loss*, and *Today's New Hypnosis* are scheduled for publication in 1997.

She is a sought-after public speaker, and television and radio personality, but thinks of herself as a teacher above all else. Her amusing, heartwarming stories linger on in the minds of her audiences long after her seminars are over.

Table of Contents

Acknowledgments

I hereby acknowledge my teachers and associates for their constant encouragement and unending support.

George Bien
Bruce Blanchette
Kendra Bond
Marie Cowden
Jeanne Engen
James Green
Sol Lewis
James Joyce
A.M. Krasner
Roger F. Meads
Richard Neves
Lee Pulos
Peter M. Rogine
Henry Smith-Rohrberg
Michael Stower
Jeffrey Ward

A special thanks to my associates and contributing editors for their constant assistance throughout the production of this book:

Norma Star Averbuck
Masud Ansari
Catherine F. Fisher
Catherine A. Hamacher
David Hamacher
Henry Leo Bolduc
Cordy Kaminski
Louis A. McCann
Kathryn L. McGlynn
Maria Reitman
Henry Smith-Rohrberg
Rita Valenti

FACILITATING WELLNESS

Foreword

From ancient times, philosophers and writers have delineated about the crucial effect of mind over body. Among others, Plato said, "We become that we contemplate." Aristotle maintained that, "Nothing is in the mind that did not pass through the senses." Einstein said, "Imagination is more important than knowledge." William James stated, "An idea, unless inhibited, tends to express itself automatically in behavior. Thoughts are associated with muscular activities." An axiom says, "Thought is action in rehearsal."

While the effect of mind over body was an established fact in the past, human beings lacked the tool of actualization of such a phenomenon, until Charcot instigated the Academia of Paris to consider hypnosis as a natural phenomenon and not as quackery. Since then, hypnosis began to flourish as an adjunct technique of medicine. During the past three decades, more research has been conducted on hypnosis than in all the preceding years since Mesmer initiated animal magnetism in mid eighteenth century. *Facilitating Wellness,* by Ms. Julie Griffin is a rarely written book in that it provides a system of structured learning.

The contents of this book will prove enlightening to anyone interested in the therapeutic arts. The reader will find the subject matter presented in a stereo form, in a clear and understandable procedure. A person interested in self-improvement and self-development can read this book with interest and intellectual gain. For those who are professionally qualified to practice hypnotherapy, the perusal of this book is genuinely didactic and self-rewarding. At the same time, it is the author's well-established experience and findings that give *Facilitating Wellness* special flavor and meaning. This book is not one initially based upon other authors' ideas to explain the research of others. Nor is it simply a recount of current literature on hypnosis and hypnotherapy. It is, rather, a sincere, objective account of the author's therapeutic successful experiences giving the novice knowledge and art, and the professional insight and confidence for propitious treatments.

Clark Hull, a prominent psychologist and a leading authority of hypnosis in 1930s, said, "An experiment without a hypothesis is blind. A hypothesis without an experiment is dead–or ought to be." In *Facilitating Wellness,* theory and practice are superbly combined. Various cases are analyzed by the author, giving the reader the theoretical epistemological insight and pragmatic expertise. Specific suggestions for each case are provided. A professional is always looking for therapeutic suggestions regarding specific psychogenic and psychosomatic disorders. *Facilitating Wellness* contains a plethora of answers to this unrespondent need of hypnotherapists.

It is my sincere opinion that everybody, whether to be a novice or professional in hypnotherapy, will find this book as interesting as I have and also will consider it of immense usefulness for therapeutic purposes.

MASUD ANSARI, B.A., M.A., Ph.D

MASUD ANSARI, B.A., M.A., Ph.D., holds a B.A. in law, a M.A. in International Relations from the University of London, and three doctorate degrees, two in political science, one from the George Washington University, and the third in hypnotherapy from the American Institute of Hypnotherapy.

He is the director of The Institute for Ethical and Clinical Hypnosis in Washington, D.C., a faculty member of the American Institute of Hypnotherapy, and author of 21 books on political science, law, philosophy, psychology, and theology.

In 1991 Dr. Ansari was the recipient of the National Guild of Hypnotists' President's Award and in 1995 he received the Eastern Institute of Hypnotherapy's President's Award. His book, *Nationalism,* won critical acclaim in 1968 and his book, *Modern Hypnosis,* is utilized as a primary textbook by hypnotherapy students worldwide.

Preface

Thirty-eight years ago my mother, June Griffin Ward, gave birth to me under the influence of hypnotic suggestion. As I grew up, my mother raved to me about the pleasant nature of my birth experience. She told me I came forth into the world without causing her any feelings other than elation and euphoria.

As a result of my joyful birth experience, I grew up with a fascination for hypnosis. I fed this fascination by taking self-hypnosis courses which enabled me to utilize hypnosis in my own life. In my exploration of the subject, I quickly discovered hypnosis was my best tool–a tool which enabled me to study and learn better, to lose weight, to quit smoking, and to overcome alcoholism. Moreover, it enhanced all my creative and athletic abilities–it helped me to dance more gracefully, to swim more competently, and to write and sing better.

Inside the knowing of the magic of hypnosis, I realized I could utilize techniques of hypnosis to give myself an edge in every avenue of my life. There came a point where I hypnotized myself prior to virtually every important thing I did. Some examples include: before job interviews, before television appearances, whenever I was in dance class or swimming, whenever I felt sick, tired, or depressed. In other words, hypnosis became a complete part of me–a programmed response to life which enabled me to achieve whatever I wanted to achieve.

It occurred to me that hypnosis was the greatest gift my mother ever gave me. As I became increasingly aware of the magnitude of this gift, I realized it was my purpose to share the gift with others–to aid others in finding the ease and comfort in their lives I have found inside myself through hypnosis. To that end, I gave up a lucrative real estate career and became a hypnotherapist.

The *American Institute of Hypnotherapy* taught me how to harness the power of hypnosis inside myself and to teach others how to harness it insides themselves. After taking the *American Institute's* basic training program, I felt as if a door to the world had been opened to me–and it truly had.

Once I went into practice, my business thrived. I established a massive group and private practice but quickly discovered my true purpose was to teach clinical hypnotherapy. It was clear to me the way I would reach the most people was to train teachers in safe, sound, an empowering methods of hypnotherapy. Now a teacher, I am aware teaching hypnosis is truly my birthright. To that end, in addition to training others in the art and science of hypnotherapy, I actively strive to educate the public through my television and radio appearances, as well as through my writing.

I would like to thank the many clients who have placed their trust in me. All the cases in this book are real but have been altered to protect the privacy of individual clients. All client's names, locations and careers have been changed. Cases selected for this text were chosen for their potential to teach the benefits of hypnosis and hypnotherapy to the public.

It is my honor to present to you *Facilitating Wellness*. I believe you will find comfort from this book and perhaps bits and pieces of your own life inside its pages. I hope *Facilitating Wellness* enables *you* to unlock your own power, magic, and love.

FACILITATING WELLNESS:
Who Am I – What Is My Job To Be?

I had my hypnotherapy certification in hand, but did it actually make me a hypnotist? How could I think for a moment I had the right or the ability to play with someone else's subconscious mind? What did it mean to be a hypnotherapist? What was I to do? How should I do it? Should I just stick to being a real estate agent and think of my certification as something accomplished out of idle curiosity? *No.*

The truth was, I was scared. I didn't know how to begin, where to start, or if I would do things correctly. I didn't even know what my job really was. I asked and answered these questions inside myself:

- Should I think of myself as a healer of minds?
  Heavens no, that was too intense.

- Perhaps I was a data entry clerk for people's brains.
  No, that was too impersonal a thought process to suit me.

- Did I want to change people? Could I change people?
  Of course not.

- So what was the point?
  I didn't have a clue.

I fumbled about with my first dozen clients. I was always nervous before they arrived, but the most amazing thing happened as they walked through my door–I instantly received the intelligence necessary to assist them. I was never at a loss for words, I was always calm.

I couldn't figure out what was happening to me. It seemed like someone was stepping into my body and asking my clients all the right questions–giving my clients all the best advice.

I noticed I frequently referred to myself as 'we' when I meant to say 'I' or 'me'. Was I going insane? Who was I talking about when I said 'we'?

For some unexplainable reason, I did not feel frightened. I realized I was getting help from an all-knowing source. The advice that came through me was always inspired, so I decided to simply be thankful for it. I wondered if this happened to other hypnotherapists or just to me. It was certainly not discussed at the certification class I attended.

It was as if I was in partnership with an invisible force–a partner who let me have all the credit. It seemed unfair. I wanted to tell everyone about the *assistance* I was receiving but I feared people would think I was crazy. For the most part I remained quiet about what was happening, but people began to ask me who I was referring to when I said 'we'. This question always startled me, because my saying 'we' was so automatic, so unconscious. Generally, I dodged the question and changed the subject as quickly as I could.

I never felt alone in my work and quickly learned I could trust the assistance coming through me. After a couple of months I determined what my job as a hypnotherapist was. **I was a *facilitator*. It was my job to *facilitate wellness*-nothing more, nothing less.** I was a vessel, a mouthpiece for information which could facilitate the wellness of others. I was comfortable with this definition; I finally had a framework inside which I could work.

It became clear to me that all I have to do is ask myself, 'How best do I help this person to facilitate his own wellness?' I am now aware this is my highest purpose–to teach others how to create their own wellness, to achieve harmony mentally and physically.

No matter what problem a client brings before me, I know his problem is only a temporary manifestation created by his being somehow in disharmony. So my job is always the same–to teach others how to achieve and maintain a state of physical and mental euphoria. Some refer to this state as enlightenment, others might call it inner-peace. But, by any name or label, it constitutes wellness. As this perfect state is achieved, whatever malady they think caused them to seek me out miraculously disappears.

I am aware now that anytime I ask for knowledge, anytime I need help, it is there. It's a wonderful feeling for which I am grateful. I have noticed that every time I help another person, I grow, and every time I help someone to heal, I heal myself.

It is a wonderful job I have–such an honor to serve in this capacity, and, personally speaking, I have never felt more happy or alive.

Waking Up
Ending Depression

"I want to tell you a story. About 15 years ago, I was very depressed. After my parents died, I couldn't get out of a blue funk. I decided I would go to a hypnotist and see if he could *make me better*. I had been overeating, drinking, smoking–I was really a mess.

When I went to see him, I was nervous because I had never gone to a hypnotist before. When I got there I was met by a wonderful man who was so full of light and energy, at first I thought he was touched in the head. He was very animated and presented himself in a way which seemed highly spiritual, although I do not believe he tried to be spiritual–this man simply was spirit. In those days I, myself, was not at all spiritually oriented.

After I told him my tale of woe, he looked at me with his eyes full of love and light, and said:

'Julie, you need to think of yourself as a living thing coming up out of the earth. Right now all you are seeing is the weeds. All you are seeing is the

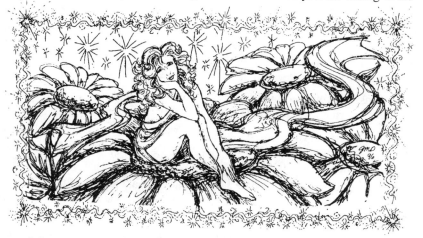

negativity. What you need to do is to picture yourself as a living thing coming up out of the earth. You need to reach down and pull out all the weeds and all the negativity which has formed around you. You need to stand up strong and tall with your head toward the sun and look for all the beauty in the world. I promise you, when you look for the beauty you will always find it. It is there; you just need to look.'

My life changed at that moment and has never been the same since. He was right; all we need to do is weed out the negativity in our lives, and look for the beauty in order to find the peace and contentment that otherwise might be lost. That advice sustained me for many years–until I came down with hepatitis A.

About four years after originally meeting him, I went to see him again. I had been suffering from chronic persistent liver disease and I figured he would be able to *make me well* again. I didn't realize in those days that all healing is self-healing. I went to see him and told him my new tale of woe:

'It began as simple hepatitis A, which should have gone away in six weeks–but it didn't. I have been running a fever for over a year. The doctors did a liver biopsy and are now calling it chronic persistent hepatitis. I don't want to be sick anymore. I am sick of being sick.'

The hypnotist seemed aggravated as I spoke of my illness. I started to wonder what happened to the loving man I had met before. Instead of speaking lovingly to me as he had the first time, he spoke in an irritated tone:

'Julie, if you are having a nightmare, and robbers and murderers are chasing you, and you see a car and the keys are in the car, do you steal the car to get away or what do you do?'

I didn't understand why he was asking me such a strange question. All I could say was, 'What?'

Again he said, 'If you are having a nightmare, and robbers and murderers are chasing you, and you see a car, and the keys are in the car, do you steal the car to get away or what do you do?'

I was still confused by the questions but I managed to say, 'I guess if it was an automatic I would steal it. I can only drive an automatic.'

He lost his patience with me and said, 'Listen to me! If you are having a nightmare, and robbers and murderers are chasing you, and you see a car, and the keys are in the car, do you steal the car to get away, or what do you do?'

I was quite upset by this time at his impatience, at the tone of his voice, as well as by my own inability to grasp the point of his question. So I said, 'I don't know what you want from me; what do you want from me?'

'I want you to *WAKE-UP!* You are having a nightmare. I want you to *WAKE-UP!*'

I was furious at him. I felt like he didn't believe I was sick. He wasn't honoring my illness. He did a hypnosis session on me after this nerve-racking confrontation, but I was too confused and angry to enjoy it. I left his office feeling very let down.

I didn't get the point of what he said until a couple months later. One day, I woke-up and realized what he meant was that I had been choosing to live inside the nightmare of illness and all I had to do was to *wake-up* from the nightmare and I would be able to heal myself. It was such a simple analogy, but for reasons I am not consciously aware of, I was not readily able to accept it. Fortunately, he planted a seed in my mind that day, and the seed grew until I understood the importance of its message.

I decided to wake-up from the illness. I actively took steps to get well. I began to drink water to flush out my system and I started eating healthfully and exercising daily. In three weeks' time, my liver function tests were normal, my fever was gone, and I was healthy. I had woken-up from the nightmare of illness that I had allowed to play itself out inside my physical body.

What I learned from these experiences with this great man, is, that we create our own realities, physically, mentally and emotionally; that we may choose to feel down, to only see the weeds; or, we can look for the beauty in the world–and find it! We can allow our physical bodies to manifest illness– or we can choose to create health inside ourselves. In other words, everything we experience is a choice.

So Candice, the point here is that I do understand that life has seemingly dealt you some bad hands. I know you have felt hurt and let down in the past, but I also know a small unconscious part of you is keeping you in the middle of the pain of the past. I know you can, over a period of time, wake-up from your sadness and hurt, and create whatever reality you want to live inside. It's all up to you now."

"I wish it were that simple," my client, Candice said.

"It will be as simple or as difficult as you make it."

I know you have been informed that you have a chemical imbalance in your body which is causing you to feel depressed, but what I want to ask you is, do you believe it?"

"I'm not sure."

"I think it is just the opposite, Candice. I think your depression is causing a chemical imbalance in your body."

"That's an interesting concept."

"Think about this for a moment. How do you feel when you fall madly in love with someone?"

"I feel great–euphoric."

"How do you feel when you work on a project which really expresses your creativity?"

"I feel the same way, euphoric, energized–like I'm high."

"Exactly."

"Now, tell me how you feel when you think about being hurt or let down."

"I feel exactly the opposite. It occurs so quickly."

"This being the case, you can see how certain thought processes instantly cause chemical shifts inside your body that make you feel good or bad. Do you see what I mean?"

"Clearly. So that is why I'm on Prozac? To compensate for the fact my depression has shifted my chemical levels?"

"Ironically, yes. I believe the Prozac does level you out, but it also keeps you in the same place. Because you are leveled out, you do not have to actively deal with your emotions. Your emotions are in limbo. You don't feel really bad, but you also don't feel good. It just becomes a cycle in which you feel numb."

"That really describes how I feel most of the time. Do you think Prozac is bad?"

"No. I feel prescription drugs like Prozac can be helpful, especially when they are being used episodically to get someone through a tough time. I just worry when someone tells me they have been on Prozac or any other mind altering drug for an extended period of time."

"Why do you worry about that?"

"Because the drugged state becomes the person's norm and can work against the person achieving his own harmony."

"Should I stop taking it?"

"Not without your doctor's permission. If you decide you want to stop taking Prozac (or any other medication), you should do so with the full knowledge and consent of your physician."

"I wonder what it would feel like to wake-up and be myself without drugs. It's a pretty scary thought. I've been taking Prozac for over a year. I don't know who I would be without it. Wouldn't I just have the screaming fits I used to have?"

"I'm not sure. Personally speaking, I'd rather have a couple of good screaming fits and really let go of the pain than carry it around with me for the rest of my life. Besides, all the things which made you want to scream happened a long time ago. I think you will be able to look at your past objectively and grow from it. I think if you go to your doctor and have him wean you off Prozac, you will be able to cope. I will do a session on you that will create the perfect mindset for you to get peacefully through the process. I

4

can also help you through hypnosis, to put the past into perspective and to move happily into your future."

"What if I decide to stay on the Prozac?"

"You may do that. It is certainly your choice. I just want you to know if you stay on Prozac it will interfere with the process you are coming to me for and it might stop the hypnosis from working completely."

"Why?"

"It's simple. The drug numbs you out and that is exactly the opposite of what I want to do for you."

"What do you want to do for me?"

"I want to help you to find yourself. I want to help you to find your own strength, love, and joy. I want to facilitate feelings in you which are so magnificent that the thought of stepping on them with a drug would seem preposterous."

"That sounds really beautiful."

"It is beautiful, and you can have it if you want to. You can decide today you are going to start a process of finding yourself, that you are going to allow yourself to feel all the joy, all the happiness the universe has to offer you, or you may stay in the state you are currently in. It's your choice."

"Do you really think I can handle life without Prozac?"

"Candice, let us stop and think about your past for a moment. Two-and-a-half years ago, you and your husband broke-up. A year later, you met someone else and a few months into that relationship, he broke-up with you. You then went into therapy and started taking Prozac. Since then, you have been in a holding pattern. Is that all correct?"

"Yes, you have the timetable right."

"Okay then, it is now more than a year after the break-up. What you have to ask yourself is, has the Prozac really helped you to start living again?"

"I guess the answer is obvious. It hasn't. If it had, I would not be sitting here with you right now."

"Exactly."

"Okay, I want to take your advice. I want to get off it."

"Candice, you don't need to make a snap decision on this. What I believe will best serve you is if we go ahead and do the hypnosis session today. I will tape the session and you may take it home and listen to it every day until you make your decision.

I believe as you listen to the tape repeatedly, it will help you bring your chemical levels back into balance naturally. It will also help you to find the courage to face your past and move peacefully into the future. Do you want to proceed this way?"

"Yes. It all makes sense."

"There is one other thing I would like to point out to you. You have been depressed for a long time. Right now your depression is a large part of your identity. I will be wording the suggestions so you can make gradual changes in your mindset. It would be absurd for me to suggest to you, 'Okay, Candice, when I snap my fingers, you will be a happy person'. I could do that, but it would not be real, and it probably would not last."

"So, what are you going to do?"

"I'm going to suggest that each day as you let go of the past, one bit at a time, you will become increasingly happy; that each day you will feel a little happier, a little healthier, and a little more excited about your life. Then, one day, after a period of time, you will completely wake-up from the nightmare of the depression you have been living with."

"I want that, Julie."

"Wonderful. In that case, it is time for you to get settled into a comfortable position. You may sit or lie down any place that looks appealing to you and I will be back with you in just a couple of moments. Feel free to begin relaxing while I step away."

I stepped out so I could clear myself. I felt certain I was about to help this lovely woman come back to life. As I walked back into my office, I felt a surge of energy moving through my body. I felt as though I was being infused with love and knowledge and embraced by the universe. Inside the office, I turned on my tape recorder and immediately began the session.

"You may allow your heart to be warmed by the realization that love and happiness are about to shine inside you and through you, and these emotions will surround you with a feeling of peaceful comfort. Notice all your muscles are becoming warm and soft, as you become aware of the peaceful feelings of love and happiness which are now moving through you.

Feel yourself going deeper into relaxation as you continue to breathe and relax. Feel your body opening up and relaxing, and opening itself, and relaxing itself.

Continue to open and relax yourself as you become aware you are developing very high self-esteem and you are beginning to feel more in control of your life and your emotions. The reason for this is because you have chosen to be happy. You have made a conscious and unconscious decision to choose joy over sadness.

No matter what may have occurred in your past and no matter how trying your past may have been, it will now be easy for you to thrive and you will delight in enjoying each moment of every day of your life.

Your heart is now being filled with love, joy, light, and laughter. You will notice you actually look better because you can see love and joy emanating from yourself. You are very aware of your breathing, and you are continuing to relax more with each breath you take, and with each sound of my voice.

Notice how easy it is to calm and relax yourself by taking in a couple of long, slow, deep breaths. You are now aware you can do this for yourself throughout the day–you can take time to breathe, relax, and center yourself. This is a wonderful, helpful skill you will utilize from now on.

I'd like you now to go to a beautiful place in your mind. It doesn't matter where you choose to go, but let it be a place of peace and comfort to you: a special place, a safe place, a secret place you know and trust inside yourself. That's right.

Feel yourself entering into this safe, peaceful, secret place, and notice the climate is perfect and that you are enjoying the peaceful stillness of your body, and the warm, glowing, love light which is radiating from your heart.

You begin to feel immersed in pleasant feelings, and for a moment you are able to let go of the past, and to let go of the future, and to discover the joy of being fully alive in the moment, alive and pleasuring inside your own peaceful wellness. It is a feeling of love, a positive feeling inside of you, and you choose to carry this feeling with you always.

Now, breathing deeply from the crown of your head all the way down to the base of your spine, you may allow all the energy centers in your body to open and resonate, as you inhale powerful forces of white light throughout your body . . . and as you exhale into warm, peaceful, relaxation . . . That's right.

Now, with all your energy centers fully open, you may allow the white light to penetrate your body, your mind, your spirit, allowing your body to glow and pulsate in a long euphoric rush of power and energy–breathing in and out deeply and continually at your own pace, as your body is pulsed and energized and healed by the loving light of the universe, and pulsed . . .and pulsed . . .

You may notice your body is being surrounded by peace, energy, love, and pleasure. Your body and mind are more alive and alert than they have ever been, even though you continue to go deeper into relaxation.

Allow your relaxation to deepen and allow yourself to experience a vast feeling of openness and a feeling of being connected into the love of the universe. Feel the power inherent in knowing you are now tied into universal knowledge and energy. Know you have the wisdom and power of the entire world at your fingertips and you will be continually tapping these resources, and you will never again feel alone.

I would like you to realize that even though things might not have occurred in the past the way you thought you wanted them to occur, that you have learned many important lessons from the various experiences you have had, and it was a combination of the good and the bad experiences which have made you who you are today–that have enabled you to wind-up right here, right now.

You may also know that you can decide to start your life all over again today–at this moment in fact. You can simply reframe the past in such a way that you may now grow from it. You may now wake-up from the nightmare of the past and find yourself embracing the future.

If there are any old feelings of despair lingering inside you, perhaps you would like to find a way to release them. Maybe you can imagine you are blowing all your despair into a balloon, and, when you decide the time is right, the balloon will simply fly away. Or, you can decide that any feelings of despair still remaining inside you are going to be slowly replaced by feelings of strength, joy, confidence, love, and courage.

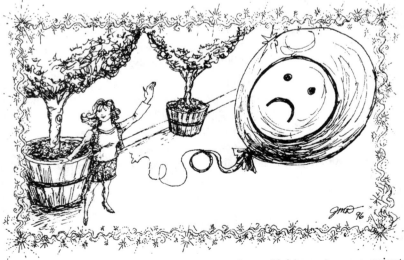

Or you can carry around your despair as if it's your own private anchor–as if it's your cross to bear. Isn't that an ugly thought?

So why not realize there is an endless well of joy inside you and it is just waiting for you to drink from it? Why not become aware you can delight in your own ability to manufacture and release joy inside yourself?

Now, as I count down from ten to one, you may allow yourself to drift and float deeper into the core of your own being and into the flow of universal energy.

> 10 - relax further into yourself;
> 9 - feel your mind expanding as your body relaxes;
> 8 - get in touch with your own essence;
> 7 - begin to release your despair;
> 6 - feel your joy filling its space;
> 5 - 4 - feel alive as you drift deeper still;
> 3 - 2 - merge with universal power and energy; and
> 1 - remain deeply relaxed and peaceful.

Now Candice you may say silently to yourself:

- I know everything I need to know to take charge of myself and I am doing so.

- I only feed myself healthy food and positive thoughts.

- I do everything with love, joy, and laughter.

- I think clearly and act in my own best interest.

- I am allowing my subconscious to work for me while I sleep, and while I am awake, to point me in the direction of my own health and happiness.

- I am allowing any feelings of doubt, fear, guilt, sadness, and negativity to leave me.

- I am moving fearlessly in the direction of my own happiness and success.

- Wonderful people are being drawn to me now that I am happier.

- I have wonderful dreams and goals set for myself.

- My body is a marvelous self-healing mechanism.

- I know that joy is a well inside of me which I may drink from always.

- I know I am the only person responsible for my health. I choose to be happy, healthy, and well.

- I turn every situation into a situation that is good for me.

- I do not allow others to mar my happiness.

FACILITATING WELLNESS

- I am very aware of my posture, facial expressions, and body language. I now use my breath to empower and relax myself.

- I stand strong and tall with my head up toward the sun.

- I do reality checks on myself often to ensure that my body language matches the words I speak.

- I speak pleasantly and optimistically to others.

- I am mentally alert, emotionally stable, and physically strong.

- I am not dependent upon alcohol, food, chemicals, or material things for happiness.

- I achieve happiness inwardly, and it shows to those around me outwardly.

- I have forgiven myself for any wrongs I have committed, and I have forgiven all others who have injured me.

- My body is growing healthier and stronger each day.

- My heart is becoming lighter and happier each day.

- I feel a glow of happiness being emitted from my heart. This glow of happiness shines through my eyes, my fingers, and my toes.

- This glow of happiness is a beacon that leads me in the direction of my health and happiness.

- This love light draws happy and healthy people into my life.

- Each day my love and joy light will shine brighter.

- I now look forward to enjoying every single moment of my life.

- My heart and soul are now pointing me in the direction of my own happiness.

Now it's time to return to full conscious awakening. You may slowly become aware of your body and breathing as you return to an awareness of the space around you. You may now return to full consciousness, fully aware that each day your capacity for love and happiness shall grow."

When Candice returned to full awakening, she seemed very relaxed and content.

"How did that feel to you?"

"It was lovely."

"You are a good subject. I'm sure this will work for you. What I want you to do is to listen to this tape for about a week and then call me and let me know what you want to do."

"Do you want me to come back in then?"

"I want you to follow your heart. Give the tape a week to work and then it will be up to you to decide what the next step will be. If you are happy with the effects of the tape, I suggest you come in to see me one or two more times. There are a few more processes we may go through to keep stepping-up the overall effectiveness of this session."

"I think I will want to proceed."

"That's fine, but you should still consider the decision over the course of the next week. That way, when you do make the choice to be happy, you will be certain it was your choice."

ONE WEEK LATER

Candice called me.

"Julie, I would like to come see you."

"How are you doing?"

"I'm terrific. It almost seems too good to be true. I stopped taking the Prozac cold turkey, three days ago, and I'm fine."

"You didn't discuss it with your doctor first?"

"No. I know you told me I should, but I felt strongly he would tell me to stay on it, and I didn't want to get into a confrontation with him. I feel too good to get into a confrontation. Besides, I've been taking his advice for over a year, and it has gotten me nowhere. It's time for me to take control of myself. I know with more of your help, I can do it."

"I'm thrilled to hear you speaking so confidently, Candice. I'm proud of you. I guess since you stopped taking it three days ago and you still feel great, you did what was right for you."

"So when may I see you?"

"How about tomorrow at nine?"

"Great."

9:00 THE NEXT MORNING

Candice arrived at my office. She was seemingly a different person than the woman whom I met the week before. Her posture was different—she stood taller. There seemed to be energy rolling off her body.

"Candice, you seem so different."

"I am different. I am really different. I feel like my old self–only better."

"What I would like to do with you today is a hypnosis experience in which you actually let go of the past. It is a powerful experience, but I think it is important. You will feel stronger afterwards. I will also give you suggestions that you will actively begin to draw love and prosperity into your life. Does that sound all right with you?"

"That sounds great."

After settling Candice in and clearing myself, I began the session. After she was *under*, I introduced the following therapy:

"You may take some time and focus on your own thoughts and become aware, in a peaceful way, of any negative thoughts or emotions you have been allowing to inhabit your heart, mind, and spirit.

Get peacefully in touch with old emotions and memories from the past which might be preventing you from loving freely and prospering now. Allow yourself to get in touch with all the old garbage, noticing how it feels physically to call up these feelings, and realize it is now time to release all the old stuff, to unload it, and to walk away from it forever.

I'm hoping you have realized you deserve love, happiness, and prosperity, and you have decided to free yourself of the limiting thoughts which have kept you from being fulfilled in the past. As a symbol of this choice, I'd like you to again focus on the feeling of weight these old hurts and negative feelings put on your physical and mental being.

Feel the ramifications of these hurts, the loneliness, and the fear of poverty. Allow yourself to feel these feelings one last time–allow them to weigh you down one last time, knowing you are about to release these feelings forever.

You realize these feelings are not serving you and that you deserve to feel the love that you are calling into yourself. You may now get ready to release the hurt, the anger, the fear, the feeling of poverty, and all limiting beliefs you have held in the past.

Now I'd like you to picture yourself in a beautiful field, and I'd like you to notice off in the distance, there is a large trash barrel with a tight fitting lid on it. I'd like you to notice as you walk closer and closer to the barrel, the weight on you is becoming more apparent, and you are becoming increasingly anxious to unload these burdens, this emotional garbage, into the trash.

As you see yourself at the barrel, I'd like you to open it, to look inside, and to mentally feel and see yourself dumping all your old garbage into it—letting go of the old stuff and feeling lighter and freer each second. Good.

Now, I would like you to put the trash barrel lid on very tightly and to walk away—free of the old garbage, free of the negative emotions, free. That was easy, wasn't it? Didn't it feel good?

I would like you also to know you have created room inside yourself for happiness. There is all kinds of room inside you that you may fill with your own love, strength, and courage.

Maybe you would like to do this but you are not quite sure how. I'd like you to know that all these things—love, joy, courage, and the ability to prosper—are already inside you. These positive traits have been there all along, just waiting for you to claim them, just waiting for you to choose them.

You may now see that everything is a choice, and now you can choose happiness over sadness—you can choose to prosper, to have every venture you engage in become fulfilling and lucrative. You can choose courage over fear, you can choose to be positive instead of allowing negativity to consume you.

Most importantly, you can choose to love, to love unconditionally, and to be loved in return—every single moment of every day of your life, starting right now by becoming your own best friend, the person who loves you the most, the person who is always there for you. That's right, you should first love yourself; it is the first step, the first movement toward creating the positive, happy, lovable, prosperous new you that you have chosen to be. That's right, engage in a love affair with yourself.

You have very high self-esteem, and you feel really in control of your life. The main reason is because you have chosen to be happy and to draw love and prosperity into your life. You have made a conscious and a subconscious decision to draw love and prosperity into yourself, and it is a wonderful choice—a choice worthy of celebration.

Although you may at one time have struggled financially, or made poor decisions in love or in financial matters, it is now easy for you to make all the right choices.

You are now drawing the right people into your life, at the right times, for all the best reasons. You are drawing in people who will love you, who will help you create prosperity, as well as people who will befriend you. You will instinctively know who you should love and who you should be friends with. You will never confuse the two.

FACILITATING WELLNESS

It will become easier for you to make the best business decisions and to handle yourself perfectly in all your business endeavors, because you now perceive yourself as a winner, and you now act like a totally successful and fulfilled person.

Every day you are becoming more confident, more self-assured, and more charismatic. People like doing business with you, and being friends with you, because of the charming, delightful, and trustworthy way you handle yourself.

Your heart is filled with love, joy, and laughter. Now, as you imagine you are looking at yourself in a mirror, I'd like you to see the happy, love-filled, successful new you that you have been dreaming of becoming.

You notice, as you look at this new reflection of yourself, you actually look better, because you now see the happy, joyous, and successful person you were always meant to be.

See how strong and tall you are standing. Observe how calmly you are breathing, and notice the beautiful smile on your face. You can see your eyes look brighter, and you are radiating love, peace, health, and confidence. What a beautiful you.

Now I'd like you to feel yourself stepping into this picture. Feel yourself filling up with love, joy, and energy. Imagine too, you can draw love, joy, and energy from the universe into yourself. Become aware you can freely share this love and energy with others, because you contain an endless supply.

You may become aware that your own magnetic qualities are increasing inside this happy new reality. Imagine you are painting your own future. Allow yourself to paint your life vividly, in beautiful colors. See yourself and your life exactly as you have always dreamed it could be. Know that you are now imagining your new mindset, your new way of being, the new you. It feels good, doesn't it? Feel the glow; feel the warmth; feel the love. These are empowering feelings you may give to yourself anytime you choose.

You are noticing there is a feeling of love and light being emitted from your heart, your eyes, your fingers, and toes, and this love light is your beacon–a beacon that points you toward happy, healthy, and fulfilling activities–the love light that draws other happy and healthy people toward you.

You are noticing that you feel free to be who you were always meant to be: a happy and fulfilled you, a healthy you. Feel exhilaration moving through you as you continue to turn up your own levels of joy and happiness.

You notice how much better the love and happiness feels compared to the former feelings of despair. You choose now to remain in the happy, positive state of self-love—choosing to remain in this love light, the love light you allowed to emerge from inside you—the love light which was kissed by universal energy.

Now, filled with joy, hope, and confidence, you may say silently to yourself:

- I choose to be happy, healthy, and well.
- I have cast away my despair and I am living my life to its fullest.
- I take time to give thanks for all I have.
- I remember to meditate or pray each day.
- I am allowing any feelings of doubt, fear, guilt, sadness, and negativity to leave me, as if all these emotions are floating away upon a cloud.
- I am allowing any talents, strengths, courage, and joy lying dormant inside my subconscious to come forward so I may use my strengths and talents, now or as appropriate.
- I am moving in the direction of my own happiness and success.
- I take time to notice the beauty in nature and all things around me.
- I remember to add music to my life, knowing that music nourishes my soul.
- Each day I take positive steps toward achieving my goals.
- My body is a marvelous self-healing mechanism. My immune system operates perfectly. I become healthier each day. My blood sugar levels remains safe and healthy.
- I achieve happiness inwardly, and it shows to those around me outwardly.
- I am free to experience unconditional love and joy.
- I have all the courage and strength I need to do anything I desire.
- I am in control of my emotions and behavior.
- I sleep well at night, and I wake-up happy and refreshed each day.
- I look forward to enjoying every single moment of my life.
- Each day I become more vivacious and charismatic.

- Interesting and helpful people are now being drawn to me because of my personal magnetism and charm.

- I have let go of old hurts from the past, and I am now free to love and to be loved.

- I realize the trials and tribulations I have experienced were actually learning experiences which have helped me to become a better, stronger person.

- I have taken on a successful, goal-directed, mindset and I am now about to prosper.

- I behave in a way that creates prosperity and I picture my success.

- I look at myself and my life objectively, and I make helpful adjustments to myself and my life.

- I am my own best friend, my own guardian angel.

- I quickly remove myself from emotionally unhealthy people and relationships. I only spend time with loving, emotionally healthy, and helpful people.

- I am whole."

As I concluded the session, I felt certain my work with Candice was completed. I gave her the tape of the second session.

"Candice, you should listen to this tape at least a couple of times, but then you may listen to whichever tape you want. I would listen to one tape or the other often, until you feel strong and happy."

"When should I come and see you again?"

"I don't think you will have to."

"But I want to. You make me feel so good. I love coming here."

"I'm glad you have enjoyed the sessions, but you need to understand that you are the one who created the happy feelings inside yourself. You may continue to do it without me. You have all the magic and strength inside yourself to keep this momentum going."

"Do you really believe that?"

"I really believe it. If you feel strongly after a few weeks that you still want to come back, I would be happy to see you, but you will not need to come back because you have already decided to be happy and to reclaim your life."

ONE MONTH LATER

I was at a shopping mall parking lot one day and I saw Candice off in the distance. Her eyes were glowing–they looked surreal. I waved to her and she moved toward me. I could see an intense energy field around her body. Light was surrounding her and being emitted from her. It was a spectacular vision to behold. Her wellness was visible.

"Hi Julie, I'm happy to see you," she said.

"You look magnificent–like you are actually glowing," I said.

"I know! I feel magnificent, too. I feel like I'm glowing. Everything is going great. I'm getting out more and having fun. I've been meeting interesting people. Thank you for changing my life."

"Thank you for allowing me to assist you, but the truth is everything you ever needed was already inside you."

Ed's Little Secret
Hypnosis for Golf

A t 5:05 p.m. my telephone rang.

"Is this the hypnotist?" the caller asked.

"Yes, this is Julie Griffin, who am I speaking to, please?"

"This is Ed Warton." *(not his real name)*

"Good morning, Mr. Warton. What may I do for you?"

"I heard about you from a friend of mine who came to you to help him run the Boston Marathon. He raved about you."

"That's nice to hear. Are you a runner, too?"

"No. I'm not actually very good at it, but I like to play golf. Do you work with golfers?"

"Yes, quite frequently. Hypnosis works beautifully for golf. In fact, every golfer I have worked with has reported back to me his friends' astonishment at how his game improved."

"I don't expect miracles, but do you think you could help me take a few strokes off my game?"

"I'm sure I can."

"So how does it work?"

"It's actually quite simple. I will have you relax and focus on your thoughts. Once you are relaxed and focused, I will have you see yourself playing better. I will have you feel in control of your game. Right now you may be intimidated by certain shots and hazards–perhaps even by some weather conditions. I can place you in the state of hypnosis, and give you suggestions that you are confident no matter what the conditions around you are."

"I don't know if I can be hypnotized. Do you think you can hypnotize me?"

"I know I can. I have never met anyone I couldn't hypnotize. In fact, you will actually be hypnotizing yourself, and I will merely be guiding you into the state."

"What do you mean?"

"All hypnosis is actually self-hypnosis. As hypnotists, we give you suggestions to help you relax, we direct you toward relaxation, but it will be up to you to allow the relaxation to occur. How deeply you become hypnotized depends on how deeply you allow yourself to relax. People usually become better at hypnosis with practice. It's just like anything else: the more you do it, the more competent you become."

"That makes sense, but are you sure I can do it?"

"We can do a simple test right now, over the phone, which will prove it. Do you want to do this test?"

"Sure."

"Okay, great. I'd like you to allow your eyes to close for a moment."

"Okay."

"Now, I'd like you to take in a deep breath . . . . and exhale . . . and imagine you are biting down on a great, big, juicy lemon. That's right, imagine you are biting down on a big, tart, juicy, yellow lemon.

Tell me honestly, did your mouth salivate or pucker when you imagined the lemon?"

"Yes, it did."

"Since you had that reaction you can be successfully hypnotized."

"How do you know?"

"You took time to focus and relax, I gave you a suggestion that you were biting down on a lemon, and your body had a physiological reaction to it. This is how hypnosis works: you relax, you focus, you receive a suggestion, and your body and mind have a reaction to the suggestion."

"That's pretty interesting."

"I agree. What we will do with hypnosis for you is to have you relax and focus, much more deeply than just now, and then I will give you suggestions which will enable you to play golf at a superior level.

What many people don't realize is that we all go into and out of hypnotic states many times a day. We do it when we are driving when we forget part of the trip; we do it when we become engrossed in a good book or a movie. Hypnosis can occur anytime a person is deeply relaxed or highly focused."

"I'm a little nervous about making a fool of myself when I'm hypnotized."

"There is no need for you to worry about such things. I am not a stage hypnotist—I am a hypnotherapist. I only use hypnosis to help people in the way they want to be helped. I will give you a suggestion early in this session that you will only accept suggestions which are truly within your highest good.

This will enable you to ignore any suggestions I make if you don't feel they are perfect for you. It will also prevent you from inadvertently accepting negative suggestions from others."

"That sounds good."

"Generally, people only accept suggestions which are within their own belief systems, but I like to protect my clients by suggesting to them they will only accept suggestions which are perfect for them. This will protect you when you hear ads on television, or if someone tries to manipulate you. It will help you long after you leave here."

"How so?"

"Again, we go lightly into a hypnotic state anytime we are relaxed or focused. When you are in this relaxed and focused state, you are far more open to accept suggestions from the outside. It is very easy for us to become relaxed and focused when we watch television or listen to the radio. Advertisers know this and use it to their advantage to get us to buy their products. The suggestion I give you about only accepting suggestions which are in your highest good will make you less of a sitting duck to advertisers and will enable you to be more selective about what messages you accept from all other walks of life."

"I like your attitude. I'd like to give this a shot. When may I come in to see you?"

"I'll mail you my intake form which I would like you to fill out and mail back to me. The form will tell me everything I need to know about you to make the session as productive as possible. I'd be happy to help you with things other than golf, if you'd like. We can work on several things in one session. You may think about it and list anything you want help with on the form. Once I get the form I will call you and set an appointment time."

"Can I make an appointment now?"

"Sure you can. I just like to be certain you are comfortable with the process before I set an appointment." I told Mr. Warton my session fee and explained it would include a tape of the session.

"I really want to do this. May I come in tomorrow? I can fill out the form when I get there so we can get right to it."

"Do you have a fax machine? I can fax you the form."

"Yes–fax it here to my office."

"I think it is a good idea for you to fill out the form before you come in because it enables you to take your time and put the proper thought into the answers."

"Okay. I'll do it. What appointment times do you have open tomorrow?"

"I can see you at 9:30 a.m. or 3:30 p.m."

"I'll take the 3:30 appointment. That will be a fun way to end my work day."

"Yes, it will. I'm sure you will enjoy it. The feeling is very relaxing and pleasurable. You will want to allow 1-1/2 hours for this first appointment because I take time to explain how hypnosis works and to teach you how to use self-hypnosis."

"How many appointments do you think I will need?"

"If you only want to work on golf, you will probably only need one appointment. Golf is simple to work on via hypnosis. I will also provide you with an audio cassette of the session so you may listen to it repeatedly at home until you achieve the results you desire."

"Wow, that sounds great. I'll fill out the form, fax it back to you, and see you tomorrow at 3:30."

"Perfect." I then gave Mr. Warton directions to my office. "Thank you for calling."

3:30 P.M. THE NEXT DAY

"Hello, Mr. Warton, may I take your coat?"

"Yes, thank you, and please call me Ed."

"Okay, Ed. How are you today?"

"I'm fine. I've really been looking forward to this."

"Please make yourself comfortable."

I took time to go through Ed's intake form with him and to briefly explain how hypnosis works.

"There is one thing I really want you to understand, Ed."

"Yes?"

"I want you to know you are the one with the magic. As you become relaxed, and as your body starts to feel good and powerful, I want you to know it is actually you creating those feelings inside yourself–not me. I want you to know that as soon as you start to practice self-hypnosis you will be able to help yourself with anything–without me."

"Do you really think I will be able to hypnotize myself?"

"I'm sure you already do it inadvertently all the time. All you need to do is take in a few deep breaths and give your body suggestions to relax. Once you feel your relaxation occurring, give your mind the suggestions which will help you to facilitate a change in yourself."

"What if I don't come out of it?"

"You will come out of it whenever you want to, just like you do when you are driving your car or watching a movie. You may tell yourself to come out of it in a specified amount of time, or you may tell yourself you will do so whenever you feel like it.

What you need to remember is that when you are hypnotized you will not be asleep or unconscious. Hypnosis is an altered state of consciousness where you are actually more aware–not less aware. At least this is true for 90 percent of the people who use hypnosis. Ten percent of the population go so deeply into hypnosis they have little or no memory of the session, but for the remaining 90 percent of us, we will consciously remember 50-100 percent of the session."

"How do I know if I fit into the 90 percent or the 10 percent?"

"It will be obvious to me today when we do the session. But in either case the hypnosis will work fine. Most people experience some of the following signs and feelings when they are hypnotized:

- you might feel warm, numb, tingly, or heavy;

- you might feel a floating sensation;

- you might feel your eyes fluttering under your closed eyelids;

- you might feel a need to swallow;

- you might feel your body suddenly jerk like it does when you are about to go to sleep;

- you will be more aware of your body and your breathing than normal;

- you will probably be more aware of the sound of my voice and of outside sounds than normal.

You will not experience all of these signs but I suspect you will feel many of them. Do you understand?"

"Yes. Do I sit-up during the session?"

"You may sit-up right where you are, or you may stretch out on the couch, or you may lie back in the recliner–whatever seems most appealing to you. Feel free to grab a blanket and pillow.

Are you sure you want to be hypnotized today?" *I always ask this question right before I begin the hypnosis induction.*

"I can't wait."

"Do you have any more questions?"

"Not that I can think of."

"Now Ed, I'd like you to breathe along with me in the beginning of this session and to imagine all the things in your mind that I suggest. This will help you to focus and relax. Once you start to relax, you don't have to pay attention to me anymore. Once you feel your body relaxing, you may allow your mind to drift and wander anywhere it wants to go. In fact, the more it drifts, the deeper you will go.

Even if you only relax slightly, you will be about twenty times more open to suggestion than you are right now. If you go into a medium or deep level of hypnosis you will be hundreds to thousands times more open to suggestion. Once again, you are in charge of how deeply you relax.

You may change your position to make yourself more comfortable at anytime during the session. You may even feel free to open your eyes during the session, if you want to. You will be in charge at all times; I will never give you a suggestion that you can't open your eyes or that you can't move. You will always be in control. Do you understand?"

"Yes."

"Okay then, to begin the process I would like you to focus your eyes up high somewhere in the room as you inhale deeply . . . and now exhale completely . . . Now you may again, with your eyes open, inhale deeply . . . and allow your eyes to close as you exhale completely . . .

You may allow your eyes to stay closed as you again breathe deeply . . . and exhale completely . . . Continue to breathe at your own pace, as slowly and as deeply as is comfortable for you, as you feel yourself relaxing more and more as you inhale . . . and letting go of stress and tension as you exhale . . . Feel all of your cells being refreshed as you inhale . . . and allow yourself to drift deeper into relaxation as you exhale . . . Very good.

Feel yourself now drifting and floating into a peaceful, euphoric place, a safe place inside yourself. That's right–find your own comfort and move freely into it. Seek out your own source and get fully in touch with your essence–the core of your being. Relax deeper now as you envision yourself at peace, as you hear your breath taking on a restful pace, as you feel your relaxation occurring and expanding. Excellent.

Imagine you are surrounded by golden, healing rays of sunshine, and these rays are relaxing your toes, your feet, your thighs. Feel warm relaxation, and golden glowing light moving into your thighs and hips, relaxing you and removing your self-doubt and insecurities as it travels through your reproductive organs and belly. Imagine you can see the golden glowing light warming and relaxing all your internal organs, your heart, your chest, and your lungs.

You may drift deeper into relaxation as you feel the golden glowing light moving into every cell, fiber, and nerve in your body. Feel it creating clear breathing passageways inside of you, feel it relaxing and energizing you simultaneously.

Notice how the glowing sunshine is traveling through your throat, into your jaw, your lips, and your mouth. Feel the warm glow traveling through your forehead, your eyes, your cheeks, relaxing the crown of your head and your entire scalp. See and feel the warm rays of sunshine moving through and relaxing your collar bones and shoulders, feel them traveling down your arms, into your elbows, and forearms. Your wrists, hands, fingers, and fingertips are all warm and relaxed now.

You can hear your heartbeat and breathing slow down as you imagine the back of your legs are relaxing; and the muscles in your hips and thighs are relaxing; and all the muscles and cells in your entire spine and back are relaxing. Notice how even the back of your head and neck are becoming warm and relaxing. Wonderful.

Now you may imagine your mind and body are opening and relaxing. As you open and relax yourself you are allowing magnificent helpful energy from the universe to travel through every cell, fiber, and nerve in your body.

That's right, just feel yourself opening and relaxing as you imagine all the colors of the rainbow are traveling through you. You may allow yourself to go deeper into relaxation with each breath you take, and with each sound of my voice.

Feel energy moving and flowing perfectly through your body, as you allow yourself to focus on all your goals, as you become aware of the fact you can do anything, and as you realize your performance on the golf course and every other avenue of your life is about to dramatically improve.

Feel your body filling up with universal energy. Feel yourself becoming energy and connecting into the flow of the entire universe. Feel yourself becoming a part of the wind which carries your ball to its desired destination. Feel yourself becoming a part of the grass beneath your feet and the club in your hands. Feel your body and mind tuning into all the conditions of the world around you–the air, the grass, the trees, the sky–knowing as you become more and more in tune with these elements you will be better able to utilize any weather or course conditions to your favor.

You will now be able to compensate perfectly for any weather or course conditions which occur wherever you are, because you can now turn any weather or course conditions to your benefit. This is because you are now a part of the wind, a part of the grass, a part of the ball as it soars through the sky, and because whenever you are golfing you are so relaxed you simply become golf.

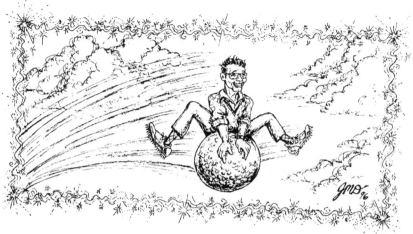

Imagine now that warm relaxation is flowing through your body. It feels nice, doesn't it? Feel the warm relaxation flowing into and out of your heart, into and out of the base of your spine, and into and out of your mind.

Feel the relaxing flow traveling through your spinal column and allow yourself to drift and float many times deeper into the pleasure and relaxation. That's right. Relax deeper as you become aware that you have infinite abilities; you have the ability to play golf perfectly and improve your game every time you play.

In this relaxed state, I would like you to focus for a few moments on a golfer whose abilities you would most like to have as your own. That's right, focus on a golfer whose abilities you would like to replicate inside yourself.

I would like you to focus more and more on this golfer and imagine you are actually entering into this golfer's energy system and consciousness. Feel yourself connecting in as you continue to open your mind and relax your body.

Now I'd like you to imagine you can actually draw the talent and abilities of this other golfer into yourself. Focus on the talent and abilities of this golfer as you become aware you will only draw into yourself the essence of this golfer's talents and abilities, and only at a level safe, helpful, and appropriate for you.

You will only replicate helpful traits. Feel yourself drawing the essence of this golfer's helpful traits into yourself . . . and feel yourself merging fully into a stream of consciousness which will enable you to replicate the talent and strengths of this golfer. Now you may feel yourself actively drawing in the talents and strengths, the helpful techniques, the style, the confidence, and any other helpful traits of this golfer. Feel yourself becoming empowered as you imagine you can actually see yourself moving around inside this golfer on a golf course. See yourself standing with the same stance, hitting the ball with the same swing, displaying a calm, comfortable, and confident manner.

Now, I'd like you to imagine you are golfing and blending your own technique and style into the parts of the technique of this golfer you would like to call your own. See and feel yourself golfing in this newly improved manner and style. Notice how great you look and feel. Fine tune the picture in your mind.

See yourself playing an entire course, in whatever conditions are at hand, knowing your game will continually improve. Feel yourself becoming more confident at each hole, with each movement, with each breath.

Feel yourself separating from the energy field and consciousness of your role model, and reintegrating into your own body, mind, and spirit. Continue to remain relaxed as you regain your awareness of the here and now.

From now on, whenever you step up to hit the ball, the only thought that will be on your mind is the thought of hitting the ball to the desired target. That's right, when you step up to the ball, you will be relaxed and focused, and the only thought on your mind will be that you can, and will, hit the ball to the target. You will perform safely and appropriately to your own highest potential. You will never exceed your body's limitations. Very good.

Now inside this pleasant and relaxed state, you may say silently to yourself:

- I have decided to perfect my golf game.
- I will be very relaxed whenever I play golf.
- When I play golf, my mind will focus on hitting the ball to the target.
- I take time to visualize the shots in my mind before making them.
- I see myself displaying the correct stance, gripping the club correctly, swinging precisely, and hitting the ball perfectly.
- I feel the air which lifts the ball and drops it where I want it to go.
- I imagine myself putting accurately.
- I see and hear the ball going into the hole.
- I feel a wonderful sensation when the ball goes into the hole.
- It gives me tremendous pleasure to visualize this process.

- I know I can practice my golf game in my mind and this process will improve my performance on the course.

- Others will be amazed at my performance on the course.

- Anytime I step onto a golf course, I automatically go into a state of highly focused relaxation, which enables me to play expertly.

- I am balanced, relaxed, and poised when golfing.

- I have perfect form.

- My mind and body connect perfectly with my golf clubs.

- I play expertly, in any and all, weather and course conditions.

- My respiration, stance, and posture are ideal.

- I eat healthfully, drink water frequently, and exercise regularly.

- I take time to relax myself several times a day.

- All the systems in my body are now balancing and perfecting themselves so that I may achieve optimum health.

- I allow the game of golf to be a pleasurable activity.

- I am aware I can improve any part of my life in the same manner that I am now actively improving my golf game.

- I am the clubs; I am the grass; I am the ball; I am the wind; I am the sky; I am golf.

- The visualization process greatly improves my mind, my body, and my game.

- Each time I see the blueness of the sky, I relax and feel renewed.

Now, Ed, you may allow all the appropriate suggestions to manifest inside your mind and body as you return to full conscious awakening, feeling alert and clear at the count of five." *I recited the count.*

"How did that feel?"

"That was great. I feel so relaxed."

"Did you feel the signs of hypnosis in your body that we discussed?"

"My hands feel like they have fallen asleep."

"Did you notice how much you were swallowing?"

"Yes."

"Were you aware of your breathing and the sound of my voice?"

"Yes, I experienced all of that."

"Ed, how long do you think the session took?"

"I don't know, maybe 10 or 15 minutes."

"Actually, it was 29 minutes."

"Wow."

"I'm telling you this because when you are hypnotized, time frequently feels a lot shorter than it actually is. You are an excellent subject, which is why it felt so much shorter than it was. You probably only remember about half of what I said to you during the session. You will realize this when you listen to the tape at home.

Do you remember the part of the session when I had you imagine you could replicate the abilities of other golfers inside you?"

"Vaguely."

"When you listen to the tape at home you will hear the part I am referring to. Each time you listen to the tape you may picture a different famous golfer and imagine you are replicating his or her best abilities in yourself and that you have the ability to blend his or her abilities with your own."

"That's wild! Will this tape make me feel the same way as the session did?"

"Absolutely. In fact you will probably relax even more when you listen to it at home because you already know what to expect. You may listen to it frequently. The more you listen to it the better it works."

"Should I listen to it every day?"

"Not necessarily. What I think would be ideal would be if you listen to it a few more times before you golf again and then listen to it whenever you want a refresher or to actively improve your performance again. But don't listen to it when you are driving or doing anything that requires your concentration, because the tape is designed to deeply relax you."

"I can certainly understand why I shouldn't listen to it in a car."

"I'm sure you will see results from this session and from the tape. If I may be of further assistance with golf, or anything else in the future, please call me. I'd appreciate it if you would tell your friends about me, too."

"I'll tell my friends who don't golf, but I'm not telling the other golfers because I want to beat them."

"This will certainly give you an edge. Thanks for coming in. You are a great subject."

TEN DAYS LATER

Ed Warton called me. He was very excited.

"Hi, Julie, it's Ed Warton. I just had to tell you I golfed for the first time this season yesterday."

"How did it go?"

"It was fabulous. It is strange, but I'm sure my stance is different and I am certain I am more confident and relaxed when I play."

"Good for you! I'm not surprised. Those are common results."

"I golfed with my usual buddies. They generally beat me mercilessly but not this time. Not only did I win the round, I won every hole."

"Great! Were your friends amazed?"

"They asked me what was going on. They suspected I had gone on a vacation and taken lessons over the winter."

"Did you tell them about the hypnosis?"

"No, it's my little secret."

"Sometimes I Talk To Cows"
Ending An Obsessive Compulsive Disorder

I was attempting to relax on a rare day off when my phone rang. "Is this the hypnotist?" a nervous voice asked at the other end of the line. *(I will refer to this caller as Mrs. Ford—not her real name.)*

"Yes, who am I speaking to please?" I asked.

The woman identified herself to me and told me a sad story about her 12-year-old daughter.

"Lisa *(not her real name)* has a disorder called trichotillomania. It's an obsessive compulsive disorder in which the person cannot resist the urge to pull out their own hair. She has already ripped out all her eyebrows and eyelashes and now she's beginning to pull out her pubic hair as it grows in. All the kids pick on her because of her lack of eyebrows and lashes.

The doctors put her on Prozac and other medications, but it isn't doing any good. All the pills are changing her personality. I told her to stop taking the pills–I want my daughter back. Can you help us?" her mother asked.

"I would certainly like to help and I believe I can help, but hypnosis depends entirely upon the client's own desire to change. If your daughter wants to be able to stop pulling her hair out, then I will be able to assist her."

"Why wouldn't she want to stop?"

"Some people feel they don't deserve to be attractive. Other people feel a desire to inflict pain upon themselves which is a form of self-hatred. I don't know why your daughter is doing this to herself."

Mrs. Ford told me a story about a school teacher pulling her daughter's hair as a disciplinary measure once. "Do you think subconsciously that has something to do with this?"

"It could possibly . . . I hope you reported the teacher to the authorities. That was certainly an inappropriate disciplinary measure."

"Yes, I called the principal."

"Mrs. Ford, I need to evaluate your daughter in person. There are many ways I can help her, but I won't know how best to do it until I see her. Once I meet with a client, I always know what to do. If I am not certain I will be able to help her, I will tell you, because I don't believe in working with a client unless I am certain of my own ability to help.

I have worked with many children. I am comfortable with kids and they always like me. I truly believe I will be able to make a connection with her and I promise you I will do everything in my power to help Lisa affect positive change in herself."

I sent Mrs. Ford an intake form for Lisa to fill out. I also wrote Lisa a handwritten note to tell her I looked forward to seeing and helping her.

I called Mrs. Ford to confirm the appointment and she still seemed nervous about the process. I took some time to explain how things would go.

"You are welcome to sit in on every session provided it is okay with Lisa. In fact, I would like you to sit in on the first session–perhaps it will relax you as well.

I think I should tell you that I am going to tell Lisa anything she tells me privately will be strictly between her and me and if she wants to see me privately she should say so. I need to establish trust with her. You need to know that if Lisa confides a personal matter to me, I will not tell you. I give children who come to see me exactly the same right to privacy as I give my adult clients," I explained.

"If I ever thought Lisa was in danger I would tell you how to intervene, but I would not disclose personal details unless it was a life threatening situation. I do this so kids will tell me things they aren't comfortable telling anyone else. Are you okay with this policy, Mrs. Ford?"

"You know, thinking back, all her doctors told me every word she said. Perhaps that is why she never felt close to them. I respect what you are saying."

"One of the reasons I tell my young clients I will not tell anyone what they tell me is because I feel, if I ever treat a child who is being abused by anyone, the child will feel safe confiding in me. I don't mean to imply I think Lisa is being abused, but you never know," I said, clarifying my position.

"If any child revealed to me they were in danger I would find a way to get the child to go to the parents or police with me. That way the child would be protected and would still trust me afterwards."

I assured Mrs. Ford both she and her daughter would be comfortable with me and we confirmed the appointment.

TWO DAYS LATER

Lisa and Mrs. Ford arrived at exactly the agreed upon time. I reached out and shook Lisa's hand (as I would an adult's) and told her I was very glad she came to see me. Lisa was tense and had not yet made eye contact with me.

I shook Mrs. Ford's hand as I motioned for them to have a seat. I went over Lisa's intake form and asked her a lot of questions. Lisa became less shy with each question.

"Lisa, how do you feel right before you pull out a hair?" I asked.

"I guess I feel nervous," she said.

"And how do you feel afterwards?"

"It's weird, because part of me feels relieved I did it and part of me feels let down I did it."

"You do want to stop doing it, don't you?"

"Yes, I do."

"Can you tell me exactly how you feel before you pull out a hair?"

Lisa thought carefully, "Yes, I feel a knot in my stomach, right here—like a nervous knot."

"Would you like to feel relaxed all the time so this knot doesn't occur in your stomach?"

Lisa nodded.

"Lisa, your mom told me the other kids pick on you. I want you to know you don't have to let other people bug you. Do you know what I do when people are bugging me? I pretend they are on the radio and I can reach up and turn them down," I said as Lisa giggled.

"Another thing you may do is imagine they are on TV and that you can change the channel. The point is, you should just ignore them."

I went on, "I wish I had known this when I was a kid because kids used to beat me up all the time. But now I have learned if someone is trying to bug me I can stop myself from hearing any of the bad stuff they are saying. I also have realized if I just smile at people they quit bugging me—it always works."

I could tell I had won Lisa's admiration. She was smiling as if in realization someone had finally told her something useful.

"Lisa, I think you are very lucky because you are learning things now about how to deal with jerks that most people never get to learn. You are going to be able to always be happy now. Isn't that great?

Plus, I'm going to give you suggestions that school work will be easier, you will be good at everything you practice, and all kinds of ultra-cool things which will make you totally awesome. Is that okay? Should we give it a try?"

Lisa was now enthusiastic. I assured her hypnosis feels good.

Lisa told me, "Everything you are saying makes a lot of sense to me."

"Lisa, is there anything else you want me to know?" *I always ask this question last, and only after I know the client is comfortable with me.*

"Yes Julie," Lisa continued, "I guess I really want you to know that sometimes I talk to cows."

"Do they ever talk back?" I asked with a straight face.

"No, but they listen to me, and I'm sure they understand what I am saying, and they care about me."

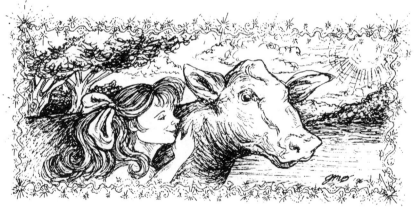

"Well sweetie, I think you should keep listening, because one of them might surprise you someday and talk back." *I said this in a serious way, because I wanted to encourage her to keep letting her feelings out—even if it was to cows.*

Lisa immediately went into a deep trance. I planted the following seeds in her subconscious:

- Now that your body is relaxed, let your subconscious register this state of relaxation so your subconscious will always work to keep your body relaxed . . . relaxed . . . relaxed—especially your stomach.

- Your hands and fingers will also remain appropriately relaxed.

- Anytime tension starts to occur in your hands, fingers, or your stomach, your subconscious mind will automatically relax these areas for you.

- If your hand ever starts to pull out a hair your subconscious mind will immediately stop it from doing so, and you will immediately forget you attempted to pull out a hair.

- You deserve to be happy and beautiful.

- You will become more creative each day.

- You will be good at everything you want to do.

- You will be so busy doing fun, healthy things that you won't have time to be nervous or bored.

- You will feel appropriately happy and relaxed.

- Every time you see the blueness of the sky you will be more in control of yourself.

- Your subconscious will seek out the reason why you pulled out your hair and it will figure out how to fix things so that you will stop.

- Every day you will be happier, more relaxed, more creative, and more popular.

- If you have trouble expressing yourself to people you can imagine, just for a moment, that they are cows, so you can speak to them easily.

I only saw Lisa twice. I made her a tape of the session and told her she could listen to it as often as she wanted. I called Lisa's mom about two weeks after the last session to see how she was.

"For the first time in a year-and-a-half I can actually see her eyebrows and eyelashes growing in. She listens to her tape every night without being told to. I can tell she looks forward to it. She seems to be her old self again," Mrs. Ford said.

Mrs. Ford added, "Julie, I want you to know that I believe in you. My little girl saw all kinds of doctors and they gave her pills and tapes and workbooks to fill out–but nothing helped. But she clicked with you. Do you know what it is you did that made the difference?"

"Yes, I acknowledged her as a person and I gave her love. Love and attention is what it all boils down to but, sadly, most people are afraid to show love or are too busy to pay attention to others. The most important thing I did, was, I gave her love. The rest of the work Lisa did herself."

I thanked Mrs. Ford for her trust in me.

A few weeks later I saw Mrs. Ford and Lisa out in public. Lisa had eyebrows and eyelashes. She was smiling and her eyes were full of light. I told her she looked beautiful and I was proud of her. She hugged me.

Love filled me.

CLARIFICATION

When interviewing a client, I always listen to what the client tells me and try to incorporate what is said into a suggestion. That is why I gave the suggestion that Lisa could imagine for a moment the people she wanted to communicate with were cows. I believe her mind made her tell me about her feelings toward cows so I would be able to use it to facilitate her wellness.

I believe when you listen with your eyes, ears, and your heart, you will *hear* your client tell you precisely what she needs.

I only worked with Lisa in person twice as she seemed to be listening to her tape regularly and it was working. I believe it would have been best to see her four to six times *(but her mother wouldn't bring her this many times because of financial concerns)*. Since finances were an issue, I invited Lisa to attend another uplifting group session I was running *(free-of-charge)* to reinforce her improved mindset.

My Friend, My Abuser, Myself
Using Regression Techniques and Self-Love to End Self-Destructive Compulsions

I was just about to leave my Brookline office when I heard the phone ring.

"Is this the hypnotist?"

"Yes. This is Julie Griffin, I am a hypnotherapist."

"This is Andrew Davis." *(not his real name)*

"Good morning, Mr. Davis. Thank you for calling. What may I help you with?"

"I'm calling about my daughter. She has a disease I doubt you have ever heard of. It's called trichotillomania."

"Mr. Davis, I'm very familiar with that compulsion. In fact, I have already worked successfully with a young girl who suffered from it."

"So you know it's a disease where the person rips out their own hair?"

"Yes. As I mentioned, I have studied it extensively and I have effectively treated it."

"Wow, this must be my lucky day. Most people have never heard of it. My daughter, Vicki, is 20-years-old. She's been ripping her hair out since she was 18. I have taken her to three different psychologists, but nothing has helped. I'm at my wits' end. It's horrifying to watch her look more and more like a cancer patient each day. I love her so much. I have to find a way to help her."

"I'm sorry for your suffering, but I do believe I will be able to help Vicki–provided she wants help."

"Why wouldn't she want help?"

"Some people have a need to inflict injury upon themselves. As long as she wants to stop, I will be able to help her."

"How will you be able to help her?"

"That will depend upon Vicki. Each client is an individual. Each individual has different motivations for their behaviors. How I assist Vicki will depend upon Vicki's motivations. So, you see, I cannot tell you how I will treat her until I have met her and discussed things with her."

"I do see; that makes sense."

"If Vicki decides she wants to see me, and you decide to bring her in, it will be fine if you want to sit in on the first session, but afterward I feel Vicki will be best served by coming in on her own. She needs to be the one who wants to come in; she needs to be the one who wants her behavior modified. Otherwise, it won't work.

During the first appointment, you may sit in during my interview and while I do the hypnosis session. That way you will have time to determine if you trust me to continue."

"I'm going to talk to her and see if she wants to meet you. I feel like I trust you already."

"Very good. I will do everything in my power to help her."

FOUR DAYS LATER

Vicki and Mr. Davis met with me at my office. After exchanging pleasantries, I read Vicki's intake form with her.

"I see you like music."

"Yes, I'm in the band. I play the drums."

"I can give suggestions which will enable you to improve your musical abilities while you are here working on the trichotillomania if you would like me to."

"Sure. That would be great."

"Vicki, do you know why you pull out your hair?"

"Well, I've thought about it a lot and I never seem to be able to come up with an answer. The more I think about it, the more I rip out my hair."

"How do you feel when you are about to pull out a hair?"

"Well, it's strange because I always feel better after I do it. I will sit around anticipating the pain of pulling out the hair, but the pain of the anticipation is always worse than the pain of actually doing it. So now I like to get the anticipation of pain out of the way by just pulling the hair out. I feel like a nervous wreck most of the time. Does that sound crazy to you?"

"No sweetie, not at all. A lot of people feel like that. When do you *not* feel like a nervous wreck?"

"I guess I feel the calmest and the best about myself when I am playing my drums or when I am teaching someone how to do something. I work a couple of hours a week at the grammar school as a teacher's aide. I feel great when I'm doing that."

"Vicki, I believe I can help you. If you'll allow me to, I'll do a session today which will relax you. I'll give you suggestions which will enable your mind to identify, in a peaceful way, why you pull out your hair.

I will also give your mind a suggestion that it realizes there is no reason good enough for it to continue making you pull out your hair. I will make suggestions which will help you to develop healthy mechanisms for everything that occurs in your life. I will also suggest that you play music and do all the things you enjoy more frequently. Does that all sound okay to you?"

"Yes, it sounds great, but do you think it will be enough to get me to stop?"

"I think it might be enough. It worked perfectly for the other girl I treated. I would like to start this way because it is the most gentle way to do the therapy. Let's work this way first. We can try more complicated techniques later if we need to, okay?"

"Sure."

"Mr. Davis, does everything sound okay to you?"

"Yes, it sounds fine."

I asked Mr. Davis to sit just outside my private session room so Vicki would have a degree of privacy. Mr. Davis was seated so he could hear every word I spoke to Vicki, but he could not physically see her.

From the position I was in, I could peer out the therapy room door and see if Mr. Davis approved of what I was saying, and I could also constantly see and monitor Vicki.

After inducing the hypnotic state through the use of progressive relaxation and creative visualization techniques, I gave the following suggestions:

- Anytime tension starts to occur in your hands, fingers, or your stomach, your subconscious mind will automatically relax these areas for you.

- If your hand ever starts to pull out a hair, your subconscious mind will immediately stop it from doing so, and you will immediately forget you attempted to pull out a hair.

- You deserve to be happy and beautiful.

- You will become more creative each day.

- You will be good at everything you want to do.

- You will busy yourself with enjoyable healthy activities.

- Every time you see the blueness of the sky you will feel more in control of yourself.

- Your subconscious will peacefully and safely seek out the reason why you pulled out your hair, and it will realize no matter what the causative factor, this behavior is inappropriate.

- If it is helpful and healing for you to consciously know the reason you have pulled out your hair in the past, you will become aware of the reason in a safe and relaxed way.

- If it is inappropriate for you to consciously know the reason why you pulled out your hair in the past, you will remain unaware of the reason.

- Your subconscious and conscious minds are now actively working in harmony to create healthy states and healthy coping mechanisms inside you.

- One day soon, you will be content.

- Your musical abilities grow each day.

- Your hands and fingers connect perfectly to your sticks and your drums as though your fingers, hands, sticks, and drums are one.

- Your soul connects perfectly to your instrument as though your soul and the instrument are one.

- You have perfect rhythm and timing, because you are rhythm and timing.

- You play music inside the flow of the universe, because you are the flow of the universe.

- Every time you hear or play music you feel relaxed and peaceful.

- Your teaching abilities steadily increase, because you are a teacher.

- You are able to eloquently express yourself in a way which delights, teaches, and entertains others.

- Every time you teach another, you learn something wonderful about yourself.

- Every day you will be happier, relaxed, creative, and increasingly popular.

I then returned Vicki to full conscious awakening by counting from one to five. As she got her things together, I spoke briefly with her father.

"She's a good subject. I'm convinced I can help her."

"I think you can, too. She seems comfortable with you. I'd like you to proceed. I believe she should see you alone from now on so she will feel free to say whatever she needs to say."

"I think that's wise. I'm glad you brought her to me. Hopefully she will only require a few sessions, but it is impossible to know until I work with her a couple times. After two or three sessions, I should be able to give an opinion as to how long this process will take."

"I don't care how long it takes. Just so long as you can get her to stop ripping out her hair. My wife and I are at a loss as to how to help her. Please help my daughter."

"I'm honored by your trust. I promise you, I will do my best."

When Vicki entered the room I handed her the audio tape of the session.

"Vicki, please listen to this daily until we see each other again. It will help you to relax, it will help your mind to identify why you pull out your hair, and it will help you to stop. Do you have any questions?"

"No, that's fine. I really liked the session. I feel better already."

"Great. Now I'd like to see you again around this time next week, okay?"

"Yes, I'd like that."

We made the appointment and I asked Vicki for a good-bye hug.

ONE WEEK LATER

Vicki showed up on time for our session. I asked her to sit in my waiting room area while I finished with a telephone call. As I finished talking to my caller, I took time to observe Vicki's body language. Vicki seemed relaxed and comfortable but I observed a hideous burn on the underside of her right arm. I concluded my telephone conversation quickly so I would be on time for our session.

"Hi, sweetie. You look pretty today. How are you?"

"I'm great! The tape really helped me to relax."

"Did it help you figure out why you were pulling out your hair?"

"No, not that I am aware of, but I don't pull out my hair much at all now."

"Really?"

"Yes, before I did it almost constantly and now I guess I only pull out four or five hairs a day."

40

"That's great! I'm proud of you. What else is going on?"

"Music class was great this week. I think your tape helped me to play better, too."

"What about your teaching?"

"I didn't have to teach this week because there was a teacher's conference, but I'm sure it will be great."

"What happened to your arm?" I said as I pointed to the burn.

"Oh, that. I work at Hardees. I burned myself on the fry machine."

"Ouch! That looks painful."

"It's not anymore."

"I'll give you a suggestion that it will heal rapidly."

"Thanks."

"Vicki, are there any other types of suggestions you want me to give you this week? I'd like to make this session different from last week's."

"No, just more of the same. Or maybe you could emphasize the relaxation. That seems to have helped the most."

"Okay, you've got it."

Vicki moved into the private therapy room and made herself comfortable. After I put on the music and dimmed the lights, she instantly went into a deep trance.

After progressively relaxing Vicki, I again asked her mind to identify the cause of her behavior and to adopt a healthy coping mechanism to the stressor that caused the hair pulling. I repeated most of the suggestions I gave her the week before and I added a suggestion that her arm would heal rapidly.

The session went well. I handed her the session's tape to take home and listen to.

"So, Vicki, it's the same deal with this tape as the last tape. Listen to this tape every day until you come in next week."

"Do I listen to this in addition to the other tape or instead of the other tape?"

"That's a good question. I suggest you listen to the new tape the first couple of days, but then you may listen to whichever tape appeals to you the most. Okay?"

"Sure, that sounds fine."

ONE WEEK LATER

When Vicki came into my office I immediately noticed a mark on her neck. As she sat down I felt compelled to ask her about the mark.

"Vicki, what happened to your neck?"

"Oh this?" she said as she pointed to the mark I was referring to.

"Yes."

"I accidentally burned it with my hair curling iron when I was doing my hair last night," she said nervously.

I was horrified because I knew she was lying. She did not have enough hair to use a curling iron. When she made-up such an incredible excuse, I knew she was lying to cover up the truth that she was burning her own body. I tried to behave normally and to not show my fear.

"How did your week go, honey?"

"It was okay. Except I am starting to remember things I don't normally think about."

"What type of things?"

"Things about my teenage years."

"What are you remembering?"

"I remember my brother used to knock me around."

"He beat you?"

"Yes."

"Do you know why he did it?"

"Yes, he did it because he was drunk and on dope. He's not really bad or anything. He's just screwed-up from being high all the time."

"How do you feel about him hitting you?"

"It's okay. He's just screwed-up. The worst thing I remember is him knocking me down a flight of stairs. I used to be really afraid of him coming home after hanging out with his friends because he would beat me up then. It's not that the beatings were terrible–actually anticipating being beaten was worse than when he actually did it."

"How did you feel afterwards?"

"I always felt better afterwards–relieved."

"Did your parents know about this?"

"I didn't tell them, but I think they suspected it. Michael was always in trouble. In fact, when he was in fourth grade he burned down the garage at our neighbor's house. Dad used to beat him with a belt to try to keep him under control but he was always bad. I didn't want to tell Dad he was hitting me because I didn't want him to get beaten. He was just a screwed-up kid."

"Vicki, I'd like you to tell me about a part of your childhood that was pleasant."

"A pleasant part?"

Vicki's face went blank.

"Yes. I'd like to understand you and your family better. Tell me about a time when you were growing up when everything was okay."

I wanted to begin the session on a positive note and to anchor Vicki to positive feelings before I proceeded to inquire about the family's maladaptive behaviors.

"Julie, I probably should have told you this before, but I don't remember much of my childhood. It is very difficult for me to remember anything before I was about eleven years old."

As Vicki told me about her memory blockage, I realized she was in very deep trouble emotionally. I knew I would have to regress her and find out what memories from the past were causing her to harm herself. I was afraid if I didn't find out what was going on immediately, she might kill herself.

"Sweetie, I think we need to do a different type of session this time."

"What do you mean?"

"If it is okay with you, I would like to hypnotize you and regress you back into your childhood so we can find out instantly what is causing you to hurt yourself. I think we need to know right now."

"Julie, you know I have been burning myself, don't you?"

"Yes, sweetheart, I know. Thank you for telling me the truth. Have you burned other parts of your body–parts I cannot see?"

"Yes, just a couple of places on my thighs."

"When did you start burning yourself?"

"About a week-and-a-half ago."

"Do you know why you do it?"

"No, Julie, I swear I don't know why."

"It's okay, Vicki, you are safe now and we are going to find out what this is all about today, and I am going to give you suggestions that you will never harm yourself again in anyway."

"Thank you. It's such a relief to know you know the truth and that you can make me stop."

"Listen to me, Vicki. We know some of the truth now, and we are about to learn more of the truth. But it is you who will get you to stop hurting yourself, not me. You are the one with all the power and I know you can do it. Do you understand what I'm saying?"

"Yes, I do."

"Do you need to tell me anything else?"

"Yes, I need to tell you I love you."

"I love you, too." *I hugged her.*

I moved Vicki into my private therapy room and got her settled. I double-checked my recording equipment because I wanted to be certain I would be able to document the session, if needed.

I induced the hypnotic state through progressive relaxation because I wanted to start the session the same way we began before. I then incorporated the following safety valve *suggestion I would be able to activate if Vicki were to incur a potentially harmful, emotionally-based, physiological response (an abreaction) as a result of things discovered during the regression.*

- "Vicki, anytime during this session you feel me tap on your forehead like this *(I demonstrated a tap in the area between her eyebrows),* you will immediately distance your emotional self from whatever you are experiencing and you will feel safe and peaceful. You will still be able to talk to me and describe anything you want to tell me, but you will feel safe and peaceful and your entire body will be relaxed."

I learned the safety valve technique from Sol Lewis, a fifty-year veteran of clinical hypnotherapy. Sol taught me it is unnecessary and clinically unsound to allow a person in trance to experience things in her mind which could unduly tax her physical body.

A suggestion frequently spoken by Sol, to prevent abreactions, as well as to aid the client in retrieving memories follows:

> "*Whenever you say the word peace or visualize the white dove of peace you actually relax. Your awareness is in control, you function beautifully, and your mind is in total recall.*"

Sol uses this phrase during regression therapy as well as when helping school children.

Once I was certain Vicki was deeply under, I regressed her back to the last day of her childhood that she could remember feeling happy. After a stated count, I asked her how old she was.

"I'm three years old."

Her manner became childlike as she spoke. She spoke as a child would speak.

"Vicki, what are you seeing?"

"Everyone looks so big. . . there is so much going on . . . it is for me . . . the presents . . . it's my birthday."

"Okay, sweetie. That's very nice. Happy birthday, Vicki. I would like you to allow the pleasant memories of this scene to remain in your mind, if appropriate and helpful. Allow your body and mind to fill itself up with happy, peaceful thoughts, and feelings of love and safety as you allow your mind to take you into a place in time you need to know about to help yourself today.

As I count from one to five, you may travel through time in a safe and peaceful way. You will be able to see the past as if you are watching yourself watch yourself on a movie screen. At the number five, you will be able to peacefully see what we need to know and you will be able to describe it to me. If at anytime during this session I gently tap you on the forehead, you will immediately feel peaceful and safe."

I had her travel on a soft, fluffy white cloud that would take her to the event for which she needed clarification as I counted from one to five.

"Vicki, tell me what you are seeing."

"It's Mommy. Mommy is mad at Vicki. Mommy is choking Vicki."

"How old is Vicki?"

I spoke of Vicki in third-person because she herself was doing so and because I believed it would help keep her distanced from any uncomfortable memories.

"Vicki is four years old."

"Why is Mommy choking Vicki?"

"Mommy is choking Vicki because Vicki is bad."

"Why is Vicki bad?"

"Vicki is bad because she got her desk messy."

"Vicki, my desk is messy, do you think you should choke me?"

"No, I would never choke you."

"Mommy should not have choked Vicki, should she?"

"No, Mommy should not have hurt Vicki."

"Vicki is a good girl, isn't she, Vicki?"

"Yes, Vicki is a good girl."

"Now, Vicki, I would like you to allow yourself as big adult Vicki to go inside this scene and save little Vicki, okay?"

"Yes, I will save her."

"Now give her a hug."

"Okay."

"Is she okay now?"

"Yes, she's okay, she's a good girl."

"Thank you big Vicki, for saving little Vicki. Now Vicki, I would like you to again travel on the white cloud to another place in time you need to know about. As I count from one to five, you may see this other time the same way you saw the last scene."

I recited the count.

"How old are you now, Vicki?"

"I'm six."

"What is going on?"

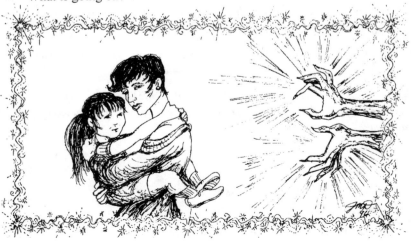

"I'm with Mommy."

"What are you and Mommy doing?"

"Mommy is telling me scary things."

Vicki became very agitated so I tapped her forehead. She relaxed a bit.

"Vicki, you are just watching a movie screen. It's okay to see what happened; you are not really there, honey."

Vicki again started referring to herself in the third person which indicated to me she was again seeing the scene in a dissociated way.

"Mommy is telling Vicki that if she is bad, monsters and the devil will get her. She said they are in the basement and she will put Vicki down there with them if she is bad. Vicki is afraid of the basement. She doesn't feel good when the door opens and she sees the stairs."

"Vicki, you know that there are no monsters or devils in basements, don't you?"

"Yes, I know that."

"Can you see that this was a bad thing for Mommy to tell you?"

"Yes, it was bad."

"And you know you are safe now?"

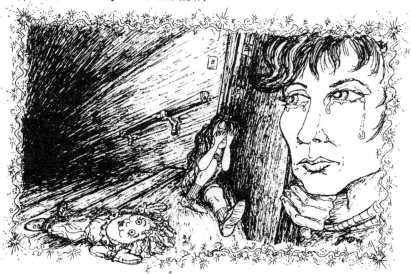

"Yes, I'm safe now. There are no monsters in the basement."

"That's right."

"I'd like you to see the picture on the screen for just another minute and I'd like you to imagine that words are being written over the screen. Okay?"

"Yes."

"I'd like you to see the words, 'the basement is safe' being written over the stairs leading to the basement. Do you see those words?"

"Yes."

"Now I'd like you to see a beautiful rainbow of color moving down the staircase, filling the basement with light and color. Can you see that?"

"Yes."

"Now I'd like you to imagine you can hear lovely, soft music coming from the basement. Can you hear it?"

"Yes, I can hear it."

"Very good. Now you can see that basements may be wonderful and realize that a basement is whatever you make it. Do you understand?"

"Yes. A basement is whatever I make it."

"Excellent. Now, I'd like you to feel the white cloud under you again. Feel yourself relaxing more and more as you allow the cloud to take you to another time you need to learn about. At the count of five, you will see another time on the movie screen you need to learn about today."

I recited the count.

"How old are you, Vicki?"

"I'm seven."

"What are you seeing now?"

"It's Daddy."

"What is Daddy doing?"

"Daddy is beating Vicki with a belt. She is a bad girl."

"What did Vicki do wrong?"

"Vicki got her party dress dirty, she is a bad girl."

"Vicki, my dress is dirty; do you think you should whip me with a belt?"

"No, I would never hurt you. You are good."

"Daddy should not have hurt Vicki, should he?"

"No. Vicki is a good girl."

"Vicki, would you send big Vicki in again, to save little Vicki?

"Yes."

"Go in and save her, and give her a hug."

"Okay."

"Vicki is a good girl, isn't she."

"Yes, Vicki is a good girl."

"Thank you big Vicki, for helping little Vicki. Big Vicki, is it all right for little Vicki to find out more about her past today? Should we keep going?"

"Yes, she needs to know more."

Whenever I am in doubt as to whether I should continue to dig deeper into a client's mind, instead of guessing, I ask the client.

"Okay then, Vicki, I would like you to again travel on the soft white cloud to another place in time you need to know about. As I count from one to five, you may see this other time the same way you saw the last scene."

I recited the count.

"Vicki, what are you seeing?"

"It's my brother, it's Michael."

"How old are you, Vicki?'

"I'm eleven."

"Where are you?"

"I'm at my house."

"Who else is there?"

"Just me and Michael."

Vicki's respiration suddenly accelerated so I tapped her forehead.

"Vicki, you may allow your body to relax, especially your breathing."

Vicki's breathing settled down for only a moment or two, and then it became even more erratic and she started screaming.

"Get off me."

Vicki thrashed about on the therapy couch as though she were trying to push someone off of her. It was clear Vicki was re-experiencing a physical attack as if it were actually occurring.

I do not believe it is necessary for someone to re-experience a horrible event as if it is actually occurring, so I immediately utilized the pressure valve technique of tapping on her forehead (again). This time, I tapped several times in a row. As I tapped on Vicki's forehead, her physiology slowly quieted down and became peaceful.

"Vicki, that's a good girl. That's right. I want you to only see the events going on like you are watching a movie of yourself watching a movie. Can you do it now? Is it okay to do it that way?"

Big Vicki's voice spoke to me rather than little Vicki's. "Yes. I'm here with her. I'll calm her down while she tells us about it."

"Thank you, big Vicki."

"Now, Vicki, continue to see it like a movie and tell me what is going on, please."

"It's Michael. He's on top of me—he's got his hands all over me. He's touching me. He's humping me."

"Was that okay with you, Vicki?"

"No, I fucking hate him. I hope he dies in Bosnia. I want him to die."

Vicki was yelling as she spoke, but her body was calm, so I decided to allow her to proceed without using the safety valve again.

"Vicki, tell your brother to get off you."

"I can't, he's bigger than me; he will just laugh at me and hit me."

"Then you may tell me what you think about him now."

"I hate his fucking guts. I want him dead. I don't want to ever see him again."

"Vicki, how old is your brother here?"

"He's 14."

"I bet big Vicki could get him to stop. What do you think?"

"Yes, big Vicki is stronger than me and bigger than him."

"Shall we ask big Vicki to make all this stop?"

"Yes."

"Big Vicki, will you go in and make him stop?"

"Yes."

"Now big Vicki, will you hug little Vicki and make her feel better?"

"Yes."

"Is that better?"

"Yes."

"Very good."

"Big Vicki, is there anything else from the past little Vicki needs to know about today to help herself?"

"No. That is all she needs to know."

"Thank you for all your help. Now Vicki, I would like you to travel safely and peacefully on the soft, fluffy white cloud, to the day you burned your own arm. On the count of five, you will see yourself as if you are watching yourself watch yourself on a movie screen. Okay?"

"Yes."

I then recited the count.

"Vicki, what are you seeing?"

"I see Vicki getting burned."

"Vicki, who is hurting Vicki is this picture?"

"Vicki is hurting Vicki."

"Vicki, is there any reason why Vicki should be hurting Vicki?"

"No, Vicki is a good girl."

"May we ask big Vicki to tell little Vicki she should be loving herself instead of hurting herself?"

"Yes."

"Big Vicki, tell little Vicki."

"Vicki, you should love yourself instead of hurting yourself."

"Now big Vicki, will you give little Vicki a hug?"

"Yes."

I watched as Vicki wrapped her arms around herself.

"Big Vicki, is little Vicki going to be all right now?"

"Yes, she is. I'll take care of her now."

"Is she a good girl?"

"Yes, she's a good girl."

"Big Vicki, are you and little Vicki the same person?"

"Yes."

"Will you and little Vicki be able to fully integrate your separate personalities into each other so you will consistently serve the highest good of your combined energies?"

"Yes."

"You may feel sensations of love and warmth surround you as you reintegrate all helpful and healing parts of yourself."

I took time to ask the last two questions and to make the last statement to be certain the experience would not inadvertently split Vicki's personality. I was comfortable after asking the questions that her mind was in touch with reality.

I then incorporated an adaptation of a procedure my associate, Henry Smith-Rohrberg, utilizes in his soul advancement therapy sessions.

"Now, Vicki, I would like you to imagine you are soaring up into a higher plane of awareness which will protect you as you see a picture of your entire life. As I count from one to five, you may allow your mind and spirit to soar into this higher plane of awareness which will help you to put the past into its proper perspective."

I recited the count from one to five.

"Now, Vicki, I would like you to understand some important things which will help you to be well and to understand your past. Is that okay?"

"Yes."

"From this plane of higher awareness, can you tell me why your mother hurt you when you were little?"

"Yes, my mother is manic depressive. She is on medication now and she never behaves like that anymore, but when I was little no one understood her problem."

"Your mother was mentally ill?"

"Yes."

"Is she nice to you now?"

"Yes, she is very nice to me now."

"Would you like to forgive her for the things she did to you when she was sick?"

"Yes, I would like to."

"Wonderful."

"Now, Vicki, you may allow your mind to think of all the things your mom did in the past which were less than perfect. You may now picture a pink light erasing all the bad images from your heart.

Do you feel that sweetie?"

"Yes."

"How does it feel?"

"It feels nice."

"Vicki, you have now created room inside your heart for more love and joy. Isn't that great?"

"Yes."

"Now Vicki, from this plane of higher awareness, can you tell me why your dad punished you when you were little?"

"It was because of Michael and my mother. Dad was having a hard time trying to keep everyone under control. My mother was always behaving strangely and my brother was always getting into trouble. My dad was just trying to keep everything from going completely crazy."

"So you think your dad punished you too much because he was afraid you would get out of control like your brother and your mother?"

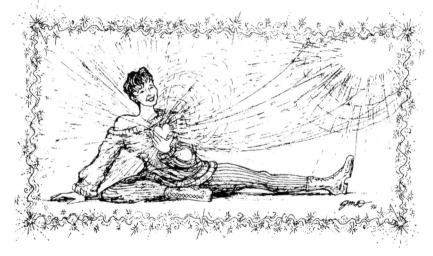

"Yes."

"Is your dad nice to you now?"

"He was always nice to me. Things were just out of control. He never got to relax."

"Your dad does seem very nice. I know he loves you because he brought you to me for help."

"Can you forgive your dad for punishing you inappropriately?"

"Yes, I already have."

"Well let's make sure your heart is healed from this too, okay?"

"Sure."

"Now Vicki, you may allow your mind to think of anything your dad did in the past which had a negative effect on you. Now picture a pink light erasing all the bad images from your heart."

"Is that okay?"

"Yes, that feels good, too."

"Very good. Vicki, from this high plane of awareness, can you tell me why your brother behaved so poorly to you?"

"Yes. It is because he is evil. He is bad, and he is evil."

"Do you know why he is evil?"

"I don't know why and I don't care why."

"Do you want to forgive him?"

"No. I will never forgive him. I hate him."

"That is okay for now. But I want to tell you something which will be easy for you to understand since you are in a high plane of awareness."

"What?"

"I want you to know that you have every right to choose to hate your brother. But I want you to understand whenever you hate someone or feel anger, it harms you more than the person you hate. I want you to know that some day soon you will be able to forgive even your brother, if you want to. If you do choose at some time to forgive your brother, there will be even more room in your heart for love and joy. Do you understand?"

"Yes, I understand, but I still hate him."

"That's okay. Just so long as you know when you are ready you will be able to let go of this hate and be filled with joy."

"I understand."

"Vicki, there is one more thing I need to ask you while you are in this high plane of awareness."

"Yes?"

"Do you know why you used to pull out your hair and burn yourself?"

"Yes, it's because I became so accustomed to feeling like I was bad and like I was about to be punished, that when I was no longer being punished by others, I started punishing myself."

"Do you know that you are a good now?"

"Yes, I know."

"So what are you going to do in the future?"

"I am going to love and protect myself."

"Very good. I'm proud of you."

I returned Vicki to a normal plane of awareness and then to full conscious awakening. As I brought her back, I suggested her mind would peacefully deal with all the information that had come to light during the session and it would develop healthy coping responses to any thought or memory the session caused to surface.

When Vicki was fully conscious, she did not remember a single word of the session. I believed the best thing to do was to tell her all the steps of the session and to tell her what she said.

"Vicki, I have this entire session on tape, but I think you should not listen to it right now. If you want to hear it later on you may, but for now I am going to keep it in the file. If you want to hear it, I will have you listen to it here with me, where I know I will be able to help you if it is difficult to listen to."

"Julie, what did I say?"

I knew it was time for Vicki to know the truth—but I felt it would be less traumatic if I told her item by item what she said, rather than having her hear herself re-experiencing it.

I recounted all the incidents of horror she experienced.

With each experience we both cried and held each other.

I told her how big Vicki had helped little Vicki each time. Her brother's sexual assault was the item most horrifying to her.

"I feel so dirty. I'm so embarrassed."

"It's not your shame to carry. You can let go of it when you want to. You told me you are not ready to forgive him and that is certainly your choice. But I gave you a suggestion that you would be able to forgive him if you ever chose to.

I'm glad you forgave your parents. I know they love you. You don't have to see your brother since he's in Bosnia. But since you live with your folks, it was good for you to be able to put this all in its proper place."

"Yes, I feel good about that. In fact, I think I remember a pink light in my heart."

"That's good. I know I usually only see you once a week, but I want to see you again tomorrow. I still want to see you a couple more times to reinforce the positive changes we've made. I know you will be okay now, but I want you to keep feeling more love for yourself and your life."

"That's good. I still want to see you, Julie."

I wanted to see Vicki the next day to make sure she was stable. I believed she would be fine, but since we unearthed so many horrible details of her past, I felt it appropriate to see her to be certain she was safely managing her emotions.

THE NEXT DAY

Vicki came in and she seemed fine but I knew my work was not finished.

"Vicki, did you tell your parents what you remembered?"

"No, I couldn't. It would hurt them too much to know that I know what they did to me."

"What is it like being in your home now?"

"It is like everyone is nervous all the time—like we are all walking on eggshells."

"Do you want it to continue to feel that way or would you like to make everything feel safe and comfortable?"

"How could I do that?"

"I think you should tell them you remembered everything and you forgave them. I think right now everyone feels responsible for you pulling out your hair. If you tell them you remember the past and you have forgiven them, you will all be able to heal from the past."

"I can't do that, Julie. I can't talk to them about this."

"That's okay honey, it was just a suggestion. I just think it is something which will put everyone at ease. But the only thing that really matters to me is that you are okay. I'm going to do another session on you to relax you and to reinforce all the positive messages I gave you yesterday. Okay?"

"Yes."

I did the session and made an appointment with Vicki for five days later.

FIVE DAYS LATER

Vicki came bouncing into my office. Her eyes were glowing with light and her entire manner seemed lighter and freer.

"Vicki, you look stunning! How are you?"

"I'm fine."

She plopped down into my big easy chair and proceeded to tell me, "Julie, I took your advice. I told my parents everything that happened here and everything I remembered."

"I'm so proud of you. How did it go?"

"It was fine. We all cried, but I told them I was going to be okay now and I had already forgiven them. Since I told them, everyone seems happier. It is like I have a normal family now. Thank you so much."

"Don't thank me, sweetheart, it was your courage that made everything right. I am so happy for you."

"Julie, I know we usually do the hypnosis now, but I have a band practice I didn't know about. Is it okay if I go now and come back for a session next week?"

"Yes, that will be just fine."

I could see there was no point in relaxing Vicki at that moment. I could not improve upon her magnificent state of mind.

"I'll see you next week."

ONE WEEK LATER

When I saw Vicki, she was still in a great frame of mind. I did another self-love and positive attitude session and sent her on her way. I told her I did not need to see her again for a month.

ONE MONTH LATER

Vicki came back in to see me. She brought me a single red rose with a card which read:

Shalom Julie,

Thank you for all your help.
I know I am okay now.

Love always,
Vicki

As we talked, she told me she had gotten a better job and a new boyfriend. She was thriving. I did a session to give suggestions she would be successful in all the important things she did for the rest of her life. I did not discuss her former hair pulling, burning, or her unfortunate childhood because I knew it was time for her to move forward—not to dwell in the past.

I knew my work was completed and her life had finally begun.

Two Cases of Trichotillomania
A Brief Comparison

I handled Vicki's trichotillomania hypnotherapy in a different way than Lisa's because, during the course of her treatment, it became obvious the treatment I used on Lisa set-off a new, more destructive compulsion in Vicki.

I don't regret beginning the therapy with Vicki the way I did, because her violent reaction to it led me to the root of her problem. I feel it is generally best to begin therapy for compulsions in the manner I chose and to use regression techniques only when they are clearly indicated.

Throughout my treatment of Vicki, I looked for similarities between these two young women which might lead me to a greater understanding of the compulsion. Since the treatment session revealed no such similarities, I decided to compare Lisa and Vicki's intake forms side-by-side.

The only similarity I observed between the girls on their intake forms *(other than the compulsion to pull out their hair)* was they both listed the same three favorite colors, in the same order. They listed the third color slightly differently, but they were describing the same color. Here is how the color lines on their intake forms read:

FROM LISA'S INTAKE FORM:

7. Please list your three favorite colors in order of preference.

1. GREEN   2. WHITE   3. MAROON

FROM VICKI'S INTAKE FORM:

7. Please list your three favorite colors in order of preference.

1. GREEN   2. WHITE   3. CRANBERRY

Although this similarity did not give me the understanding of trichotillomania I was hoping for, it did alert me to the possibility that color plays a role in health and in healing.

Since I made this connection, I now consistently incorporate color-related healing suggestions when working with clients. Four examples follows:

- You may now see your imbalance as a color.

- You may actively draw a second color into the imbalance that will bring your body, mind, and spirit into a state of balance and harmony.

- You may now see and feel a third color moving through your energy system which represents health and harmony.

- You will now actively continue to draw into yourself the proper light and colors which will balance and perfect you.

I have no statistics to support the fact that the above technique has merit, but I feel strongly it does and I shall continue to use it and to look for connections between color and healing.

The most important reason these two young women required completely different therapies for the same presenting problem is because they are two completely different people. Alas, there is no exact procedure or formula for hypnosis which will work at all times for all clients. Each client must be treated as an individual, because each client is an individual.

Thwarting Those Pesky Mosquitoes
Creating Internal Insect Repellent

A mother called me and asked me if I could help her child. "We are here on vacation at the lake, and my seven-year-old daughter, April, is getting horribly bitten by mosquitoes and deerflies. I have been spraying her with organic insect repellent because I'm afraid to put chemical repellents on her. Even when I do spray the repellent on her, she keeps going swimming and washing it off."

She continued, "She seems to be allergic to the bites. They swell up, itch, and drive her crazy at night. I took her to a pharmacist who suggested an antihistamine salve to stop the itching, but she is still very uncomfortable. Can you help her to feel more comfortable? This is ruining our vacation."

"Yes, I'm sure I can help. You may bring her in this afternoon if it's convenient." We set-up a time for April to come in with her mom.

April, her mom, and her sister Maylin, arrived on time. When I saw April, it was obvious her mom had not exaggerated her child's condition. There were visible insect bites all over her body which were swollen and had scabbed over from her scratching. Maylin had a few bites here and there on her body, but they were not swollen and itchy like April's.

"Hi, kids," I said to them as they bounded into my office.

The children seemed very excited to be in my office. They both really wanted to be hypnotized.

I told their mom I could hypnotize both of them simultaneously, even though it was only April who was having a problem.

"I'd be happy to hypnotize both the girls. During the session, April will get suggestions that will help her with the bites and she and Maylin will both get suggestions that will help them with their school work and to build self-esteem. I will only charge you for one session, but, since they are both here, I might as well assist both of them. All the suggestions I make will help both of them."

"Can we, Mom, please?" Maylin asked.

"Sure, if it's all right with Julie, it's fine with me," the mother said, sounding pleased by my suggestion.

I explained how hypnosis works in simple terms and I asked them where they would like to travel in their minds during the session. Much to my surprise the girls wanted to go on an African jungle safari. I told them I would take them on a jungle safari during which they would receive magical healing powers. They were both very happy to participate.

After their mom filled out and signed the intake questionnaire and release form, I asked April and Maylin to sign it, too, so they would feel important.

"Okay, girls, I need you both to sign this form right under where your mom signed it."

The girls both did as instructed.

"Now you two may sit or lie down wherever looks most comfortable to you, and prepare to go on a safari."

"Mom, are you going on the safari, too?" April asked.

"No, I don't think so," her mom said.

"You can be hypnotized, too, if you'd like, or you may just watch them. It makes no difference to me," I said to the mother.

"I think I'll just sit over here and watch them," she said.

"Very well," I said.

"Okay girls, are you ready to go?"

"Yes," they both said.

I dimmed the lights and turned on the music which sounded the most safari-like from my collection. To induce the hypnotic state I had the girls process the following:

- ♦ I instructed the girls to imagine they were on a hammock and that the hammock was rocking back and forth.

- ♦ I had them imagine as the hammock rocked them back and forth, their bodies were relaxing more and more.

- ♦ I had them imagine the sun was shining brightly and warming their bodies from head to toe as they continued to swing back and forth.

- ♦ I had them imagine their bodies felt like they were melting into relaxation.

- ♦ I told them as they continued to swing on the hammock they would feel their breathing relaxing their bodies, and with each breath they took they would go deeper into relaxation.

When I could see by the girls' facial expressions and hear by their breathing that they had entered the hypnotic state, I had the girls imagine the hammock was turning into a magic carpet and that they were safely flying to Africa for the safari.

"That's right. Feel the hammock now turning into a beautiful, safe magic carpet. Feel yourself flying to Africa. Imagine you can look down from the magic carpet and see how beautiful the world beneath you truly is.

Now, I'd like you to imagine the carpet is landing in Africa. That's right, I'd like you to see yourself on a safari in Africa. You are riding on the back of an elephant, up high, feeling safe and sound. You may look around and see monkeys waving to you from the trees, and lions and tigers running through the jungle.

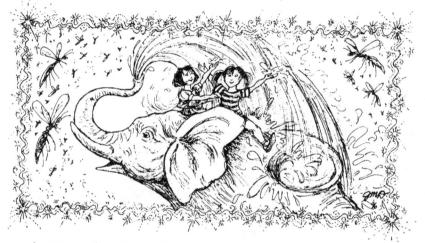

As you continue to ride through the jungle on the elephant's back, you notice how different people look in the jungle and how beautiful everyone and everything is. Then you hear your tour guide make an announcement. You can hear her saying through the loudspeaker:

'Attention all safari people. We are now approaching the pool of healing. This is a very special pool that heals your body. No matter what is happening inside or outside your body, this pool will make your body function perfectly and feel great. This pool will give you the magic ability to heal yourself in the future.'

As your elephant comes to a full stop you notice there are a couple of cute jungle boys there to help you climb down from it.

You notice how warm your body feels and you look forward to going into the pool of healing. You look at your mom and dad and they tell you it is okay to swim in the pool of healing.

Quickly you jump into the pool and notice how good the water feels against your body. You notice the water is bubbling and its temperature is perfect.

Now as you enjoy the feeling of the water moving around your body you may become aware that the water is healing every part of your body, especially the parts of your body that have been bitten by bugs. That's right, your whole body is being healed–especially your bug bites.

Next the tour guide comes over and tells you the water has other magical abilities.

'All the children who swim in this water become smarter,' she continues, 'they all find it easier to study and learn after they have been in this pool.'

You may continue imagining you are swimming or wading in the pool of healing knowing as I count from one to ten your entire body will begin to feel perfect. *(I recited the count.)*

Okay kids, it's time to return to America now. I'd like you to picture yourselves drying off and getting back on the magic carpet which will take you home.

Feel yourselves sitting on the carpet and buckling up your carpet belts. Feel yourself becoming smarter as the carpet takes off. Imagine you are looking down and waving good-bye to the jungle boys, the tour guide, and all the beautiful animals. Notice how great your body feels as you fly home to America. It is a very fast trip because magic carpets fly very fast.

Now, I'd like you to picture yourself back at the lake. I'd like you to imagine your body is making a chemical which keeps bugs away. That's right, imagine there is a tiny little factory inside you which creates the perfect, healthy chemicals that makes all bugs want to stay away from you. As I count from one to five, I'd like you to feel yourself creating the healthy chemicals inside your bodies which will keep bugs away from you. *(I recited the count.)* Very good.

I'd also like you to know, now that you have swum inside the pool of healing, your body will remain comfortable throughout the rest of this vacation and always. Your body will remain comfortable unless your mind needs to give you a warning signal. You will continue to feel any warning signals necessary for your protection. Your health will be perfect because your body creates its own health.

It will now be easy for you to study and learn. You will even enjoy the subjects that used to seem hard because they will now seem easy and fun. You will see a pattern in everything you are learning which will make learning pleasurable.

All your creative and musical abilities are becoming enhanced. You will be able to draw, paint, write stories or poems, sing, dance, become an athlete, or anything else your heart desires.

You will enjoy eating healthy foods and practicing all the things you want to become good at. Each day you will feel happier, healthier, more relaxed, more creative, and confident. It will be easy for you to talk to your parents, teachers, and all the other important people in your life.

You will instinctively know who you should be friends with and who you should stay away from. You will always think clearly and act in your own best interest.

You know you are as good as anyone else and that all people are created equal. People will like you because you are a nice person and because you treat everyone the way you like to be treated.

You sleep well at night and you wake-up happy and refreshed each day. You look forward to enjoying every moment of every day of your life. You have the ability to grow-up and become anything you want to be. Excellent.

Now, at the count of five, you may return to full conscious awakening, remembering what it's like to be on an African safari and knowing you feel great and that the bugs are going to stay away from you."

As I recited the count, the girls returned full of energy and ready to describe the animals they saw, and what it was like to ride on an elephant and to wade in the pool of health.

Their mom winked a wink of approval at me as she wrote out a check for my fee.

"I made them a tape of this session, but I don't think they will need to listen to it. If they want to listen to it they may, but it is not necessary. Kids are excellent hypnosis subjects and I believe this session has already accomplished everything we set out to do."

"They certainly seemed to enjoy it. It was fun to watch them. Thanks for putting in the suggestions about school and self-esteem. I really appreciate all your trouble."

"It was no trouble. It was a honor and a pleasure to assist you all. Have a great vacation."

THREE DAYS LATER

On the last day of April and Maylin's vacation, I heard from their mother.

"Julie, this is Kathryn Halloway, April and Maylin's mom. I just want you to know I haven't seen April scratch herself even once since we left you, and I really believe the girls did not get bitten after they left your office. I wanted to say thanks again, but I also want to know what chemical the body produces to repel mosquitoes."

"That is a very good question, Kathryn. Unfortunately, I do not have an answer for you. I have never even heard of that therapy before I tried it on the girls. My original intention was just to get the bites to stop itching, but all of a sudden the idea rushed through my head. I realized that there could not be any harm in suggesting it, so I did. I'm glad it worked."

"It really did work. I'm amazed. But I'm still curious."

"What are you curious about?"

"I'm wondering why it worked since there isn't really a chemical in the body which repels mosquitoes."

"I didn't say there wasn't such a chemical, I just said I didn't know of any."

"So there might actually be such a chemical?"

"Probably. I think the human body has an innate ability to generate any chemical needed to ensure its own survival. I have successfully assisted clients with depression by suggesting they achieve a chemical balance inside their bodies that makes them feel good."

"So this is the same sort of thing?"

"It could be, but there are many different theories pertaining to occurrences such as this. For example:

- the body tends to create anything the mind can imagine;
- all the cells in the human body act as receivers and carry out the orders sent to them by the subconscious and conscious minds;
- we create our own realities with our beliefs; and
- whatever we fully believe, we will automatically manifest.

So the truth is, I don't know why April's skin stopped itching or why the girls stopped getting bitten. It could be because they changed the chemical levels in their bodies by using the powers of their minds; it could be because they believed they were healed in the magic pool of healing; or perhaps their minds sent their cells a message to create a state change inside their bodies."

"That's a lot to ponder. I didn't realize so much thought goes into the process of hypnosis."

"What I do is, I make a wide variety of suggestions and allow the suggestions which are most appropriate for the client to manifest in a way that best serves the client. I don't feel a need to know exactly why something worked, I just need to trust that something I say will work."

"Whatever happened, it saved our vacation and more importantly it made my daughter more comfortable. I want you to know I am truly amazed at how well this worked."

So was I.

The Penis Man
Effectively Treating Sexual Dysfunction

Yes, I know–the title of this chapter is shocking. I know I shouldn't refer to a client as *The Penis Man*, but perhaps, as I begin at the beginning and allow this story to unfold, you will understand why I think of this client as *The Penis Man*.

Ned Stone, *(not his real name)* called me on the phone one day after reading an article about me in *EARTH STAR*, a holistic health magazine.

"Hello, is this Ms. Griffin?" he asked.

"Yes, how may I help you?"

"Well, this is kind of embarrassing, but I was wondering if you do sex therapy and how many sessions I would need to get well?"

"That all depends, Mr. Stone. I do sex therapy, but I only accept cases I feel comfortable with. I am unable to tell you precisely how many sessions you will require because how quickly you get well depends on how good a hypnotic subject you are and how frequently you listen to the reinforcement tape I provide. Most of my clients only require one appointment."

"Just one appointment?"

"Yes, it's because I tape the session and you are then able to hear it over and over again. I will also teach you how to hypnotize yourself so you can help yourself when you are not with me."

"How do I know if you will take my case?"

"I will mail you an intake form which allows you to put into writing the nature of your condition. The form asks specific questions and allows you to elaborate on your condition comfortably. Once you mail the form back to me, I will call you so we can discuss your condition, and decide if it's appropriate to meet. Does that sound okay?"

"Yes, it sounds very good. I think writing about my condition will be much easier than talking about it."

"All my clients like using the form. It prevents embarrassment. I do want you to know there is no need for embarrassment. I am here to assist you and I feel it is just as important to help people with sexual maladies as it is to work on conditions like asthma or weight loss."

"I appreciate your saying that. You can mail me the form at . . . ."
he proceeded to give me his mailing address.

SEVERAL DAYS LATER

I received Ned Stone's intake form with a tell-all letter attached to it. The pivotal issues and comments from the letter and the intake questionnaire follow:

- I have dreams about being tied-up and sexually toyed with. I don't know if this is normal.

- I feel like a failure with my girlfriend because I have not had an erection in over a month.

- I want to please my girlfriend and provide her with a good erection and powerful orgasms.

- I want to be able to have powerful orgasms when she wants me to.

- My girlfriend wants to tie me up and penetrate me anally with dildos. I don't know if this is normal.

- I'm afraid of not being able to satisfy her needs and desires.

- I'm afraid I will never have an erection again.

After reading the letter, I carefully checked the intake form to see if my client was on any medications which could prevent him from obtaining an erection. *(Certain medications, such as blood pressure medication and anti-depressants may have a detrimental effect on sex drive.)* My client was not taking any medications at all.

Next, I checked to see if the client smoked, drank heavily, or used illicit drugs. *(Smoking, alcohol, and drug use may all have detrimental effects on sex drive.)* My client stated in writing that he did not smoke, hardly ever drank, and was drug free.

I then checked to see if he exercised regularly and ate healthfully. *(Regular exercise and a healthy diet may increase sex drive.)* The form indicated he exercised frequently and had a health-conscious diet.

As I read Ned's letter and intake form I felt I was dealing with a psychologically- or emotionally-based problem. It also occurred to me it was possible my client was not achieving an erection because he did not want his girlfriend to tie him up and penetrate him anally with a dildo.

I decided to take this case because I felt I would be able to assist Ned and because nothing on his intake form felt threatening to me. I called him to make the appointment.

"Ned, this is Julie Griffin."

"Yes, Julie?"

"I've read over your form and I'd be happy to see you if you still want to proceed with an appointment."

"Yes, I do. Can you see me tomorrow? I'm anxious to do this."

"Sure, that will be fine. Is 4:00 p.m. okay?"

"Yes, that's great. How should I dress? I'm a salesman and I usually wear a suit and tie. Is that okay?"

"Sure, you may wear whatever you want. In fact, a lot of people wear sweatsuits or gym clothes so they will be comfortable."

"That sounds better. I guess I will plan on going to the gym after I see you, so I will go home before our appointment and change into my gym clothes."

"That will be fine. It really doesn't matter. If you don't have time to change, you may simply take off your tie and loosen your collar. I can assure you, you will be perfectly comfortable in my office."

We discussed the fee and reconfirmed the appointment time.

4:00 P.M. – THE NEXT DAY

Ned Stone arrived roughly on time for his appointment. He entered my office wearing a T-shirt and silky-looking gym shorts. He appeared nervous and avoided making eye contact with me. I reached out and shook his hand and asked him to be seated.

"Thanks for coming to see me, Ned. How are you today?"

"I'm fine . . . but I'm a little nervous about this."

"It's natural to be nervous. The session will be relaxing and you'll leave here knowing you can control your body. I'm here to help you learn how to control your body. You may start to relax now."

I took time to go through Ned's intake questionnaire with him.

"Ned, in your letter you asked me a few questions and I want to go through this information with you. Is that okay?"

"Yes."

I addressed and phrased all comments in a clinical manner.

"Ned, how long has it been since you were able to obtain an erection?"

"I guess it has been about a month."

"How long ago was it that your girlfriend decided she wanted to tie you up and use a dildo on you?"

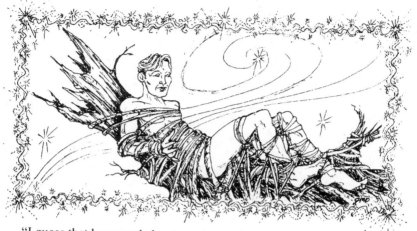

"I guess that happened about a month ago, too."

"Ned, is it possible you are not having erections because you don't want your girlfriend to do that to you?"

"Yes, I think it's possible. Part of me wants to do it to please her, but mostly I think it's pretty weird. Is that normal?"

"Whatever two people agree they want to do together is normal and natural, provided it is not physically or emotionally harmful to either of them and provided they both truly want to do it. For example, there is nothing wrong with your girlfriend wanting to do that to you, but there is also nothing wrong with the fact you don't want her to. Do you understand what I mean?"

Ned looked relieved.

"Yes, I'm glad you said that because I don't want to feel like she's weird or like I'm weird."

"Is she pressuring you to do this?"

"She really wants me to let her do it. She says I will get used to the idea and eventually I will go along with it. She has been sticking her fingers up there trying to get me ready for bigger things."

"Do you enjoy that?"

"No, not really."

"Why do you allow her to do something to you that you do not enjoy?"

"I want to make her happy."

"Do you want to get used to the idea?"

"I don't know."

"Ned, once again, there is nothing wrong with her wanting to do it, but there is also nothing wrong with your not wanting her to do it. What is inappropriate is her attempting to coerce you into doing something you do not naturally want to do."

"I see."

"It might be that you are not sexually compatible."

"But I love her."

"I understand, but sexual freedom and enrichment only occur when both parties are able to happily express and meet each others desires. There are times when peoples' desires are not compatible. That is not anyone's fault. You should examine all of this carefully and decide if this relationship is appropriate for both of you. It is important you openly discuss how you truly feel with your partner–that way you will be able to find out if there is a way you can meet each other's desires in a comfortable, compatible way.

You need to understand that I will not be giving you a suggestion that you will want her to tie you up and do this to you because I will never give you a suggestion regarding sexuality that is not naturally within your nature or spectrum of desires. So if you are here because you want me to make that seem appealing to you, I must tell you that I will not do that because it would be a violation of your true nature."

"Then how can you help me?"

"I can give you suggestions that:

- your body functions perfectly;

- all the chemical, hormonal and blood pressure levels in your body are balancing themselves healthfully so you can fully enjoy your sexuality and achieve optimum health;

- you are able to achieve erections and orgasms at will;

- you are a wonderful lover and partner;

- you are able to please your lover in a way which is comfortable and appropriate to your own needs and desires;

- you are able to communicate perfectly with your girlfriend and all other people in your life;

- you have a healthy attitude toward your body and your sexuality and you are able to express your sexuality freely; and,

◆   you will be able to let go of any sexual taboos which are not appropriate for you which were put into effect inside you due to religious or social programming.

Those are the types of suggestions I believe will help.   Did all the suggestions sound okay to you?"

"Yes, all those suggestions sound helpful."

"If you would like, I can also put in suggestions regarding sales persuasion."

"I would appreciate that very much."

As is my custom at the beginning of each private session, I explained to Ned how hypnosis works and I asked him if he had any questions.   I also explained to him what it feels like to be hypnotized and all the sensations he might experience during the session.

I went on to explain to Ned that all hypnosis is actually self-hypnosis. All he would need to do would be to follow my suggestions and, after a few long, slow, deep breaths, he would be able to find himself entering into a pleasantly relaxed state.   I also told him he would be in control throughout the session and he should only allow his mind to accept suggestions which were truly within his own highest good.

I told Ned he would be able to use this same process on himself at home, or any other place, anytime he wanted to focus his attention or to relax himself.   I told him that after he listened to the tape a few times, he would be able to remember how to relax and give himself suggestions without the tape.

"Ned, is there anything else you want me to know?"

"No, I don't think so."

"Are you sure you want to be hypnotized today?"   *(I always ask the client this question one last time, right before I begin the process.   It's a good way to show you respect the client's desires.)*

"Yes, I'm sure."

"Okay, great.   You may remain seated or you may lie down."

"Is it all right if I stretch out on the couch?"

"Yes, I think you will be very comfortable that way.   Would you like a blanket or sheet to cover yourself?"

"No, I'm fine."

"Ned, I'm going to step out for a minute.   You may allow yourself to relax to the music–I'll be right back to start the session."

CLEARING PROCEDURE

I went into the restroom and did the ritualistic things I always do before I begin a session. 1) I gargled with mouthwash to clear my voice and to make certain my breath was fresh; 2) I washed my hands; 3) I took a few deep breaths to clear myself and to draw universal energy through my body; 4) I asked the universe to guide me through the session; and 5) I asked the universe to protect me and my client during the session.

This clearing procedure is a vital component of any session I facilitate. During the procedure I temporarily divorce my own ego so I can become a vessel for pure and helpful universal energy and knowledge. Once this procedure is put into effect, my own physical energy system is bypassed and universal energy fills me. This prevents me from passing any of my own *stuff* to the client, as well as from picking-up my client's *stuff*. By creating this state inside myself, I safeguard my own energy system and provide my client with a pure form of universal energy. I also find that during the clearing process I automatically achieve a trance state which is perfect for maintaining focus.

I returned to my office, turned on my recorder, and began the session. I had Ned focus his eyes on the ceiling while breathing deeply to induce the trance state. After a few deep breaths I instructed Ned to close his eyes and to allow relaxation to grow and spread throughout his body. I gave suggestions that all his energy centers *(chakras)* were opening, resonating, and pulsating, and that energy would continue to flow freely through him.

I had the client imagine the color red was moving through the base of his spine and allowing any remaining tension in his body to disappear.

Next, I had him imagine the color orange moving through his reproductive organs, which would enable him to have powerful erections and orgasms, and would allow his passion to emerge.

I then had him imagine the color green moving through his heart and that, as he felt the color green moving through his heart, he could forgive himself for anything he did wrong in the past, and he could forgive anyone who wronged or injured him in the past. I suggested he was free to give and receive unconditional love and to enjoy his sexuality.

Next, I had him imagine the color blue moving through his throat. I suggested this to enable him to communicate his needs openly and freely to his lover, in a way which would make his lover want to respond to his needs. I also gave him a suggestion that he would be able to communicate perfectly with his clients, and that his sales persuasion would dramatically increase.

I suggested he see the color indigo moving through the space between his eyebrows *(his third eye region)*. I told him as he pictured this, his intuition would increase, safely, to a degree which would enable him to know how best to function in the world around him.

Finally, I had him picture a wonderful violet colored light shining into the crown of his head enabling him to get in touch with his own highest truths and feelings of power and control.

At this point, I observed my client's penis dancing around inside his shorts. It was going up and down, and up and down, and flying around. His penis seemed to have taken on a life of its own. It was disturbing to watch, so I shifted my gaze elsewhere and continued to give the therapy suggestions.

After a few minutes, I looked back at Ned to make sure his breathing was stable and his body responses were normal. At that time, I was shocked to realize he had taken his penis out of his pants and placed it snugly in his hand.

It's difficult to know what to do at a time like this. I felt like I was in the middle of a hypnotist's nightmare. It seemed as though all different parts of me were having conversations with each other.

- Part of me just wanted to run out of the office and leave Ned.

- Part of me wanted to give him a suggestion to put his penis back in his shorts.

- Part of me reminded me that I couldn't give him the suggestion to put his penis back in his shorts because it would ruin the audio cassette I was making. *Why?* Because the client would feel embarrassed each time he played it.

- Part of me wondered if he would ejaculate all over my couch.

- Part of me feared that if he did ejaculate, it would fly over and hit me.

- Part of me feared the situation would get even more out of hand *(no pun intended)* and the client would make a physical move on me.

I silently gave myself the following suggestions to put myself back in control of the unfortunate situation.

- You are a therapist.

- You will manage this situation perfectly.

- You will remain calm throughout the rest of this session.

Once I gave myself the above suggestions, I realized what should be done. I positively anchored Ned to the fact he was having an erection–therefore he could! I gave the following suggestions:

- You are now fully aware you can obtain an erection.

- You are aware of the feeling of an erection.

- You are aware of the sensations of the erection.

- You are aware of the chemical balance in your body when you have an erection.

- You may now allow your subconscious to register this chemical balance and all other sensations in your body.

- You will now be able to instruct your subconscious to recreate this state inside you whenever you wish to achieve an erection and an orgasm.

- Your subconscious will automatically create this state of excitement, and chemical and hormonal balance anytime you want to have an erection and orgasm.

- That's right, you are aware you have an erection and that you can recreate it anytime you desire.

I was not touching Ned in any way at anytime during this session. I believed the above technique would anchor him effectively because he was touching himself while the suggestions were given.

I would never suggest a client touch himself sexually, but since he already was, I incorporated it into the therapy. After giving these suggestions, I concluded the session as quickly as I could.

I was nervous about concluding the session because I knew when Ned returned to full consciousness he would realize his penis was in his hand. I feared that, since he was such a deep subject, he might think I made him do it.

I did my usual arousal technique *(again, no pun intended)* counting up from one to five. As I counted, I looked away from the client and grabbed the audio cassette I made of the session. I thought I should take it into my outer office and dub it for my files in case I ever had to prove I did not give him a suggestion to touch himself.

As I walked out of the room with the tape I said, "Ned, I'm going to give you a few minutes to pull yourself together. I'll be back in a short while."

Ned made a primal sounding noise when he became aware of the fact that his penis was in his hand. I kept walking.

When I started dubbing the tape, my whole body was shaking. I quickly realized I did not want to wait the ten minutes necessary to dub the tape; I wanted to get the client to leave my office as soon as possible. I concluded it was extremely unlikely a male client would sue me for what occurred because he would be too embarrassed. I also realized when Ned listened to the tape he would know I didn't do anything wrong.

I took a deep breath and reminded myself that I would say all the right things when I went back into the office with Ned. I quickly decided to speak to him in the same manner I speak to any client after a session. I had to behave as if nothing unusual had occurred.

When I walked into the room, Ned was sitting on the couch waiting for me.

"So, Ned, how are you doing?"

"I'm okay."

"Did you feel comfortable throughout the session?"

"Yes, but I feel really stupid right now."

"There is no reason for you to feel that way. You needed help and you came here and got help. You can feel proud of yourself for having the courage to get the help you wanted. Besides, the session was very successful."

"It was?"

"Yes, I'm sure of it. What I want you to do is go home and listen to the tape very carefully, while you are fully alert. I want you to become consciously aware of everything I said during the session."

"You mean you want me to listen to it while I am awake?"

"Yes, just the first time. I think you were so deeply hypnotized during the session you may not remember what I said to you. I think it is important you know consciously all that I said. After you listen to it once, consciously, you may listen to it whenever you want and let yourself go deeply into trance again. Do you understand?"

"How many times should I listen to it?"

"You may listen to it whenever you want to, but I think you will probably want to listen to it once a day for about the next week or two to help your mind fully register and accept the suggestions you want to accept."

"Okay. Do I need to see you again?"

"Probably not. I think this session will be enough, provided you use the tape as I suggested."

"Should I call you and let you know how I am doing?"

"You may if you would like to, but you don't have to. I am sure you will be fine."

Ned got up and started to leave my office.

I quickly stopped him because he had neglected to pay my fee. "Ned, will that be cash or check?"

"Oh yeah . . ." he said as he pulled out his wallet, "cash, how much was it again?"

I told him my fee, but as it turned out, he was $15.00 short of the amount agreed upon. "That's okay, I will bill you for the rest. Here is a receipt. Thank you for coming in. Drive carefully."

When Ned left I called my faculty advisor, Dr. Richard Neves, at the *American Institute of Hypnotherapy*, to discuss what had occurred.

"Dr. Neves, it's Julie Griffin. You won't believe what just happened during my session." I proceeded to tell him the story. I felt like I needed to get it off my chest.

"Julie, you shouldn't have let the guy take his penis out of his pants."

"I didn't let him. His penis was jerking around in his pants so much I looked away so I wouldn't be distracted. When I looked back, it was out."

"Did you anchor him to the erection?"

"Yes, I did." I said, and I went into detail on how I proceeded.

"I guess you handled it the best way you could in a bad situation."

I felt relieved my advisor hadn't yelled at me. I felt relieved the entire event was over.

The next day, as I thought the session over in my mind, I realized I should not allow it to prevent me from treating other sexually related cases. After all, nothing like this had happened before and, as uncomfortable as it was, I managed it professionally and I believed I helped him affect the desired change.

CLARIFICATIONS

In all the years I have practiced sexual enrichment therapy, I have never had anything else like this occur before.

My client was in a very deep trance and I believe his behavior was an automatic response to the arousal he felt, as a result of the sudden resonance of his energy centers.

I did not think he did this on purpose or to 'give me a show'.

EPILOGUE

About a month later, a colleague of mine called to tell me she had treated a client for sexual enrichment and the client had left the session without paying her fee.

"What exactly did he come to you for?" I asked.

"He came to me because his girlfriend left him because he could not achieve an orgasm."

I immediately suspected her client was Ned Stone.

"Can you tell me more about your client?"

"Yes, he said he's a salesman. It was kind of strange, when he called he asked me if he could wear shorts to the session. Isn't it a little cold for someone to want to wear shorts?"

"Did anything unusual happen during the session?"

"What do you mean?"

"Did he get an obvious erection or start touching himself?"

"No, nothing like that. It was just a normal session. I did a lot of research and spent two hours with the guy and he walked out without paying."

"Why didn't you stop him?"

"I did, I said, 'That will be $120.00'."

"What did he say?"

"He said, 'Oh, I thought you would bill me.'

I said, 'No, I expect to be paid now.'

He asked, 'Do you take credit cards? I don't have money or a checkbook with me.'

I told him, 'No, but there is a cash machine right across the street. Please go over there, and get the money and come right back with it because my next appointment will be here in 15 minutes.'

He said he would, but he never came back. I'm furious about it. I've called him at home and at work. When I called the sales office where he said he works, they said they never have heard of him."

"I have to ask you," I said, "was his name Ned Stone?"

"Yes, how did you know?"

I proceeded to tell her my Ned Stone story.

She was horrified.

"That's it! I'm not taking any other sex cases. I don't think you should either," she said.

"I have already taken other sex cases. I thought Ned Stone was on the level. Now it sounds like he is a weirdo getting thrills at our expense. But I'm not going to let one weirdo stop me from helping people who are on the level."

"I think we should call the police and report him."

"You can't. He is your client and you are supposed to keep your clients' names confidential. Technically, we should not have discussed his name. The only reason I did was for our protection."

"He's not really a client because he didn't pay me."

"Yes, he is a client, because you treated him. Once you accepted him into your office and actually treated him, he became a client whose rights you are supposed to respect."

"Even though he didn't respect my rights?"

"I'm afraid so. My best advice to you is to just let go of this. Learn from it and let go of it."

"I'm going to make everyone pay in advance from now on. I spend a lot of time preparing for a session. I can't afford to not get paid when I invest all my time and energy."

"That's your decision, but I know I will never do that."

"Why not?"

"Because I would be insulted if anyone I went to for help asked me to pay in advance. Besides, if someone trusts me to hypnotize him, I feel I should trust that person to pay me. Even if I get stiffed a few times, I'm not going to waste energy being concerned about it, because I know my conscious is clean, my karma is good, and the universe will provide me with everything I need. That's really all I need to know."

"So, you are going to leave yourself wide open to idiots like Stone to take advantage of your nature?"

"No, actually, this experience has opened my eyes a bit. From now on I am going to verify my client's place of employment before treating sexually oriented cases. I want to make sure that the client gives me a legitimate name. It has always been my practice to give my secretary my client's name and phone number for security reasons. Now I will also verify the client's place of employment. Beyond that, I am going to leave such things in the hands of the universe."

So my friends and associates, now you know why I call him, **The Penis Man.**

Richie's Escape From Autism

Richie, age five, was not just a client; he is also my handsome little nephew. Richie was trapped inside a disorder most commonly know as autism. No one knows exactly what causes autism or what goes on inside the minds of the autistic. No one knows what causes the autistic to hide inside themselves—what scares them.

While I knew taking the case of a relative was a risky thing to do, I felt no other therapist would work harder to free Richie of his disability than I would—no other therapist would care as much as I do.

To complicate matters, I lived 1500 miles away from my nephew. The distance seemed, at first, to be a huge obstacle toward successful ongoing treatment. Fortunately, it did not turn out to be an obstacle at all.

My sister was at her wits' end as to how to help her son. She sought the advice of many *experts*. She questioned her doctors as to what possible value hypnosis might provide. The experts told her hypnosis wouldn't work because her son's biggest difficulty was his inability to process language at a sufficient level. In other words, hypnosis would not work because Richie could not talk. Fortunately, my sister ignored them.

It was true that Richie's verbal communication skills were severely delayed. At age five, he had approximately the same verbal skill level as his spunky two-and-a-half-year-old sister. While observing him, it struck me that although he had trouble speaking, he possessed his own unique intelligence and was capable of listening. Even though he frequently seemed to be in his own world, I believed I would be able to *reach* him.

My sister constantly worried about one of Richie's habits. Richie *pouched* food. He would leave a small amount of food in his mouth at the end of a meal for hours. This behavior alarmed my sister and caused her to live in constant fear that Richie would choke to death. She forced him to swallow his food, but moments later he would discreetly regurgitate it back into his mouth. A specialist said Richie's holding food in his mouth was a security gesture; other kids had security blankets to hold onto—Richie had partially decomposed food.

The specialist suggested my sister give Richie something else to chew on—something too large to be swallowed, like a rubber ball with a string tied to it—claiming this had helped other kids with similar problems. I knew this was not a solution. I didn't want any child to go through life with a rubber ball in his mouth—it was simply unacceptable.

I observed my sister plead to her son to swallow his food. "Please Richie, I'm afraid you will choke on your food–please swallow it for Mommy." I noticed her words, "you will choke," seemed to actually cause Richie tension. The fear of choking seemed to be causing tension to occur in Richie's jaw. The more he heard it, the more he needed to keep the food in his mouth to help diminish the tension.

My first session with Richie was in August 1992. It seemed as though Richie knew why I was there. He seemed to have an extraordinary sense of my purpose, even though no one had discussed it with him and despite the fact he was not consciously aware I am a hypnotherapist. Richie sat down with me, in the comfort of his own home, as though he knew it was time for him to start freeing himself from his affliction.

I was nervous about treating him prior to my arrival, but suddenly I felt as if all the right words were coming out of my mouth. I felt a comfortable, peaceful feeling sweep through me. I knew I would do and say all the right things–because I had to.

It occurred to me that Richie might appreciate being spoken to like an adult–most kids enjoy this. I've learned children appreciate it when you are direct with them about their difficulties (provided you don't dwell on them).

As Richie quietly fixed his eyes on a toy on his lap, I took a deep breath and said, "Richie, I bet it really bothers you that you can't talk like your friends."

Richie immediately looked up. He seemed gratified someone had finally acknowledged his problem and relieved I wasn't protecting him from the reality of his situation. Instead, I faced it squarely with him, in a loving manner.

"Do you know what?" I asked. "It will be very easy for you to talk when you do just a few simple things."

I had Richie's full attention.

"As far as I can tell, there are only two silly reasons why you can't talk and I believe you can easily fix both of them." I didn't wait for him to respond, but rather, told him what he needed to do.

"First you have to learn to relax . . . relax . . . relax, especially your mouth and jaw." *I spoke to him playfully as I lightly ran the tip of my fingers across his jaw and asked him to relax.*

"It is easy to relax. All you have to do to relax is laugh. Another way to relax is to breathe deeply *(I demonstrated what I wanted him to do)* and if you breathe deeply just three times a day you will always be relaxed–

especially your jaw. *(I lightly stroked his jaw again.)* I bet you can feel your jaw relaxing now.

Another thing which will relax you is if your mommy or daddy strokes your hands with their fingers *(I demonstrated it to him)*. Anytime your mommy or daddy does this to your hand, your whole body will relax.

It will be very easy for you to talk when you stay relaxed and when you spit the food out of your mouth. Just stay relaxed and spit the food out of your mouth and you will be able to talk as well as your friends."

At this point, my sister, who had been nervously waiting in the hall, joined us. Richie, without coaxing, ran into the bathroom and spit the food he had in his mouth into the toilet. My sister appeared amazed.

"I'm really impressed," she said.

Seconds later Richie was back in the room, talking in nearly complete sentences, and was obviously proud of his ability to do so.

I took Richie aside a couple of hours later, and told him I was proud of him, and repeated all the suggestions I had given earlier in a playful way. I added a suggestion that soon his desire to hold food in his mouth would disappear.

I had attended Ernest Telkemeyer's workshop on telepathic trancing and aura-stroking at the *National Guild of Hypnotists' Convention* just the day before. I decided I had nothing to lose by utilizing Mr. Telkemeyer's procedure on Richie. I was behind him and it was easy to stroke his aura downward as Mr. Telkemeyer had suggested. It had a relaxing affect on Richie and it appeared to make him feel good.

As I watched his relaxation blossom, I held my fingertips on his wrist. I felt a mild sensation, like a faint electric current, move through my fingers into his wrist.

I telepathically sent him messages such as, you will remain relaxed, everything will be easy now, you can talk very well, you can control your body perfectly, you can make yourself comfortable any place or anytime, and, you are always peaceful.

As I *transmitted* these messages, I was amazed by Richie's stillness. He was usually unable to sit still. It seemed as though the transmission of suggestions made him feel as good as it made me feel. It seemed like the procedure had worked.

A couple days later, Richie was sleeping on the couch beside his dad. As he slept, I quietly sat next to him and transmitted suggestions to him again. As I lightly touched his wrist, he began to awaken, but as he realized I was with him, he drifted back to sleep. In a moment, I observed his eyes roll back under his eyelids which were slightly open. I noticed his nose and lip twitch sporadically–he was clearly in trance.

I telepathically transmitted the same suggestions as the day before. Afterwards, I suggested his trance would turn into normal sleep and that he would wake-up when he had slept sufficiently.

I contemplated how I could explain the telepathic trancing to my sister without her thinking I lost my marbles. Finally, after playing it over in my mind, I decided I would just tell her the unedited truth.

I couldn't tell what was going on in her mind as I gave her the details of my sessions with Richie. Fortunately, she didn't seem stressed by it.

"It occurs to me that Richie is intensely telepathic. There seems to be no harm in communicating with him this way. I believe this type of communication will work best for him. You can learn to work with him this way, too."

"I couldn't. I'd be too afraid," she said.

I explained that all she had to do was to be certain of her son's ability to become totally functional.

"You need to be certain–you need to have positive thoughts only. You need to mentally send him love and encouragement every single day. I'm afraid what has been happening is, as you worry about him he mentally picks up on your fears, and it makes his problems worse."

I explained to her *(as nicely as I could)* that, when she phrased things negatively *(for example: I'm afraid you will choke)* she caused nervousness in her child. "You need to give him a positive reason for spitting the food out instead of a negative reason. Next time, try saying, 'Richie, as soon as you spit the food out of your mouth, you will be able to talk to mommy.'"

She agreed to try phrasing things positively, and she acknowledged the logic in what I said. I told her I felt uncomfortable correcting her because I thought she was the best mom on the face of the earth. She told me I should never feel bad about telling someone the truth, as I was capable of doing it in a loving and helpful way.

I didn't see Richie again for four months, but my sister gave me regular progress reports. "I can't thank you enough," she continued, "Richie almost never pouches food anymore, but if he does, all I need to do is tell him that if he wants to talk to me, he should spit the food out of his mouth. It always works. My life is so much easier now that I don't spend every moment wondering if my son is about to choke to death. Even if no other change comes from this hypnosis, you have given me a great gift already."

"Much more will come of this," I assured her. "It's just a matter of time. I know Richie will be well–he is supposed to be well. Please continue to send him this message mentally."

Late in December, I saw Richie again. I was amazed at how well he spoke. His manner also seemed improved. His eyes appeared brighter and he made eye contact with others more readily.

"Richie, I am so proud of how well you can talk now," I told him.

"Aunt Julie, I spit out now," he said.

I was amazed he had remembered my giving him this suggestion and by the fact that it was clear he wanted me to know it helped him.

My heart was singing; I had made a difference. I felt a lump form in my throat as I said a silent thank you to whoever gave me the knowledge to help Richie affect change in himself.

On this visit, I only worked with Richie telepathically. I waited until he was sleeping and I held onto his wrist and sent more positive suggestions. I made the suggestions more complicated because I knew he was ready for them. I sent the following suggestions:

- You will continue to make progress.

- Your mind will identify what is holding you back and your mind will make it right so that you are not held back anymore.

- You can control your body.

- If your clothes feel bad against your skin, you may tell your skin to feel nice. *(This suggestion countered his over-sensitivity to the feeling of clothing against his skin.)*

- Every time you get on the school bus, you relax.

- Every time you get to school, you relax.

- Every time you go home, you relax.

- Every time you see the sky, you relax.

I mentally gave him dozens of suggestions, like these, in a repetitive manner. As I mentally spoke to him, I imagined his wellness in my mind; I visualized his relaxation; I saw him as a totally functional child and adult.

As I gave him messages, I could see many indications that he was in trance. His eyes were rolled back and his eyelids were one-third open. His mouth and nose twitched sporadically. His throat pulsated. He was making pleasant cooing noises throughout. Occasionally he giggled.

I motioned to my sister to come and sit next to me and I proceeded to point out all these indicators to her while Richie remained in trance.

After arousing Richie, I took my sister aside and explained to her what I had pointed out. "Those were all trance indicators. This procedure is perfect for him; his response is obvious. I want you to start doing this with him every day."

"I'm afraid I will do it wrong. I don't know if I can do it," she said, expressing her concern.

"You can't do this wrong. All you need to do is mentally send love and encouragement. You can't do it wrong. You don't even need to touch him—just continually send him love and encouragement and, most importantly, you need to know in your own mind that your son is about to thrive. If you have any doubts, they might telepathically transmit to Richie."

"It all makes sense," she told me, "but I guess I still don't believe I can do this just because you can."

"There is nothing special about me except I have given myself the courage to use this procedure. As soon as you give yourself the courage to attempt it, you will be able to do it."

I reminded her of the many times she and I had experienced telepathic occurrences between us when we were growing up.

"This is the same thing, except you will be doing it purposefully. I know you can do it—anyone can do it."

Shortly after I returned home, I received a letter from my sister. She told me she dreamt Richie was locked in a dark prison and the only way should could communicate with him was through telepathy. In the dream, she had the courage to do so. In the dream, she sent him the right mental messages until a light appeared and he was set free. As her son was freed, she heard a voice telling him he could now go and help the others. She told me that despite the fact this experience occurred during her sleep, it did not feel like a dream.

"It was too intense, too real to have been a dream. It was obviously a message for me. I know he is going to be okay soon. He is going to free himself. I'm going to start communicating with him telepathically—I know I can do it now," she wrote.

I called her after I received the letter and she told me anytime she sent him the mental message, "I love you Richie; I'm proud of you; you are fine," he would run to her, hug her, and tell her he loved her, too.

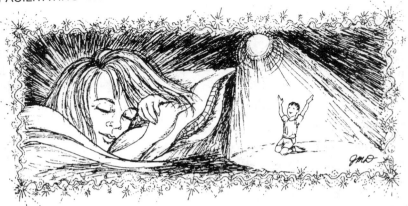

"It's amazing," she said. "I have tested this frequently, and I even do it from behind him so he can't see my facial expressions, yet he consistently acknowledges the love and encouragement I send him. This is wonderful."

My whole body glowed as she continued to tell me, "Since you left, I have seen at least a twenty percent improvement in his overall condition. Thank you."

I was so choked-up it was difficult to speak, but I finally managed to say, "Thank you for trusting me and for having the courage to help him in this manner. You will be able to help him constantly now. This will be a time for his rapid improvement. I will continue to see his condition improving in my mind, too."

I thanked the heavens and felt blessed to have been able to facilitate such a magnificent occurrence.

SUMMARY

At age six Richie entered a regular public school's first grade class. He continues in the public school system with the help of an aide. Although many of Richie's mannerisms are different from his peers, he is frequently perceived as a *normal* child. Richie has friends, a regular schedule, and is progressing by leaps and bounds daily.

In sharing this story, the point I most want to impress upon you is that I had no idea whether these techniques would work when I first used them. I let a combination of my learned knowledge and intuition guide me. I weighed out the possible benefits and risks of these techniques and I decided no harm could come from their use.

So, I encourage others who have clients with uncommon difficulties to use alternative methods (provided they could only have a healing effect should they work).

If I hadn't had the courage to try these alternative methods, my nephew might still be sitting in a corner, staring at the wall.

Going The Distance
Creating a Marathon Mindset

"Hello, may I speak to Julie Griffin, please?"

"This is Julie Griffin."

"Hi, my name is George Farrington. (*Not his real name.*) I was referred to you by Maria Lazarro. She told me you specialize in athletic hypnosis."

"Specialize is a strong word. I am very good with hypnosis for athletics because I use it myself, and because it is a passion of mine, but actually I have a general hypnotherapy practice."

"How do you use hypnosis athletically?"

"I am a long distance swimmer. I can put myself in a trance and swim indefinitely."

"Is that safe?"

"The way I do it, it is. I give myself suggestions to train properly, eat healthfully, and that my body will function perfectly. Beyond that, I suggest that I will perform up to my highest capacity while remaining respectful of my body's needs and warning signs. This prevents me from going into a mindset which could endanger me physically."

"That sounds very appropriate."

"I also use hypnosis for dancing. I have studied ballet and jazz for over 15 years and recently have started to tap. The hypnosis increases my fluidity and creativity as a dancer, and it also helps me to remember dance routines."

"Wow! Have you worked with runners before?"

"Yes, I have."

"How would you help me? I've run two other marathons unsuccessfully. Both times I crapped out around mile 17."

"I will suggest you train properly, eat healthfully, drink water, and, most importantly, that you see yourself crossing the finish line. I will have you visualize yourself running the course peacefully, and I will have you see yourself crossing the finish line. Once you process these suggestions, it will become probable in your mind instead of seeming impossible."

"That sounds helpful."

Those are the most important seeds I will be suggesting to your subconscious if you come in. I'll also tape the session for your use."

"Great. I'd like to make an appointment."

FIVE DAYS LATER

George Farrington arrived at my office 15 minutes late.

"I'm sorry I'm late, Julie. Parking is hell in this neighborhood."

As George settled in, I quickly reviewed his intake form.

"George, you seem to be pretty well adjusted. I've never seen an intake questionnaire so absent of concerns, yet something is telling me you are having trouble sleeping at night. Is that true?"

"How did you know?"

"I don't know how I knew. Intuition, I guess. You didn't check the box on the form for sleeplessness, but a little voice in my head said I should ask you."

"That's amazing."

"Yes, it is. I guess it comes with the job. So, tell me about the sleep problem."

"It's not a big deal. That's probably why I didn't check it off on the form. I just have trouble sleeping about half the time."

"George, do I have your permission to help you with that, too? Your being well-rested will help your training program."

"Sure. That will be great."

"Okay then . . .". I proceeded to explain how hypnosis works and to teach George how to hypnotize himself. Afterward, I asked him to make himself comfortable so we could begin the session.

"George, would it be okay if I touch your arm and forehead during this session? It will help me to cue your subconscious."

"Yes, that's fine."

I had George breathe along with me and visualize his body relaxing more with each breath. Once he started to relax, I moved into the focus of the session.

"Allow your body to relax completely, as you imagine yourself running on a course toward your higher awareness. That's right, find yourself on a safe path to your own truth–the truth which will free and empower you.

As I count from one to five, I would like you to feel increasingly relaxed."

I recited the count.

"Anytime you feel me gently squeeze your wrist you will relax more and move further into higher awareness."

I squeezed his wrist three times in a row and continued to squeeze it at varying intervals throughout the session.

"George, I would like you to know you are capable of anything and you have unlimited abilities. All you need to do to run a marathon (or anything else in your life) is the following: create the correct mindset; be certain of your own success; prepare for your success appropriately; and take the necessary steps toward the fulfillment of your goal.

To create the perfect mindset, I would like you to see yourself getting psyched for the marathon. Imagine yourself establishing a proper training schedule.

- See and feel yourself sleeping soundly at night. It will now be very easy for you to fall asleep at night. As soon as you get into bed, you will take a few long, slow, deep breaths, and on or before the seventh deep breath, you will drift into a natural state of sleep. You will sleep soundly at night, only waking when it is appropriate. The quality of your sleep will be profound. You will wake each day at the correct time, and you will notice you awaken feeling happy and rested.

- See yourself eating healthfully and drinking plenty of water.

- See yourself correctly fueling your body with the food and water which will create a storage room of energy inside you.

- Imagine you can see and feel yourself running just the right amount each day so you build the proper physical endurance level which will ensure your completing the marathon.

Now, I'd like you to create the marathon in your mind. That's right, it's marathon day. You are in Hopkinton at the starting line. You feel confident of your ability to reach the finish line. You are excited by the reality of what you are about to accomplish. You are enjoying the presence of the crowd and the camaraderie you feel with the other runners. You take time to properly prepare yourself just before the race. Perhaps that means eating or drinking something in particular; or perhaps it means warming up your body by stretching; or perhaps it means getting into the proper focused mindset. Picture and feel yourself making all the right motions to ensure your success. Very good.

Imagine now you are hearing the starter's signal. As you start running you notice how well conditioned your body feels. You allow your body to go into a state in which it perfectly paces your internal and external functions. That's right; your body is starting a pacing system inside itself. It will automatically regulate your breathing, your movements, and every function inside itself to ensure your health and safety during this event.

Picture yourself remaining comfortable during the run. Imagine you are at mile five, and you are feeling strong and confident. You are now at mile ten, and you notice you are just as comfortable as you were at mile five. Suddenly you find yourself at mile 13, and you realize you are half-way to the finish line. You notice your body is performing and regulating itself perfectly for your comfort.

Now you realize you have passed the 18 mile mark. That's right, you made it well beyond the point where you used to stop. You know now that you are going to go the entire distance, because you successfully moved through the 17th mile. As you feel me tap your forehead, you will become fully aware of the fact that you can go the full distance."

I tapped his forehead.

"There are now only three miles left. A wonderful feeling of euphoria seems to be carrying you. You know you are running, but it feels like a power greater than yourself is moving you forward. You are happy that there are so many people at the sidelines cheering you onward. You notice how wonderful the positive energy of the crowd feels."

I tapped his forehead.

"As you move into the city, the pleasure in your mind and body escalates. You feel a wonderful, helpful surge of adrenaline and endorphins moving through you. As you run through Kenmore Square, the sound and size of the crowd quadruples. You use the sounds of the crowd's cheers to move you toward the Prudential Center."

I tapped his forehead.

"Suddenly you are there, crossing the finish line. Now, when you feel me tap your forehead, your mind will fully register yourself crossing the finish line (*I tapped his forehead*). Feel how proud you feel of yourself (*I tapped his forehead*). Realize your body performed perfectly for you during the run (*I tapped his forehead*).

You know this is the result you desire and deserve, and that it will be easy for you to create it in reality, because you will sleep soundly at night, (*I tapped his forehead*), eat healthfully before the race and always (*I tapped his forehead*), train correctly (*I tapped his forehead*), and perceive yourself as a success.

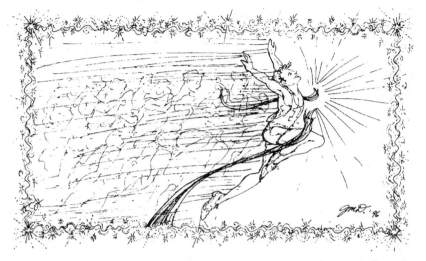

George, you are now aware you are capable of completing the marathon. You may allow this marathon mindset to carry through into all other areas of your life because there are many important finish lines in life which have nothing to do with running.

That's right, you will be able to set goals for virtually anything, knowing you will take all the right steps toward their manifestation. You have developed a knowing of your own ability to be, do, have, or become anything. Isn't it a great feeling?

Allow your heart and mind to silently speak these words along with me:

- I will complete the marathon safely.
- I will train properly for this event.
- I will eat healthfully and drink an appropriate amount of water.
- I will continually visualize my success.
- I will continually imagine my body regulating itself.
- I will perform up to my highest potential–but I will be mindful to honor the warning systems and needs of my body.
- I will pay attention to and respond properly to any warning signs my body provides.
- I feel universal energy empower me when I run.
- I will make it to all the important finish lines in life."

I then suggested George return to full conscious awakening.

"Wow. That seemed so real."

"It was real because anything your mind creates has it's own *real* energy. Your mind has registered it as though it has already occurred. That is why you will now be able to perceive yourself as capable of completing the run–because you already have. The more you listen to this tape, the more you will reaffirm it as your reality."

"You taped it?"

"Yes, here it is. It's for you to keep. Feel free to copy it for your friends."

"Wow. I'm really grateful."

"I appreciate your allowing me to assist you. I'd love to hear about your success after the race. Will you call me?"

FIVE WEEKS LATER

George called.

"Julie, I made it! It was just like the tape. I was relaxed, I felt high, and my body performed excellently. I was tired and sore afterwards, but I think that comes along with running 26 miles."

"Sure it does. I'm glad you called, and that you made it to the finish line. Congratulations. I'm very proud of you."

"The only thing is, I should have made copies of the tape."

"Why?"

"Because my buddies and I were fighting over who would get to hear the tape one last time in Hopkinton. I felt guilty about keeping it for myself."

Getting To The Root of the Problem
Attempted Suicide

I had never dealt with a client who had attempted to take her own life before. I had no experience in this realm. I was uncomfortable with the thought that if I failed to reach this client she might actually kill herself.

Nancy *(not her real name)* had been referred to me by her sister. I had already successfully treated five other members of Nancy's family *(for varying problems)* so naturally they were all counting on me to save Nancy from herself.

The trust the family placed in me weighed heavily on my shoulders. I did not want this responsibility but I felt somehow I would receive the guidance I needed to facilitate Nancy's wellness. To make matters worse, Nancy was from out-of-town. I would only have one appointment with her. It was a make-or-break situation if ever I had been in one. I had to affect a change and I had to do it immediately or she might die. I cleared my calendar so I could give Nancy a double-length appointment.

As is my custom, I had Nancy fill out an intake form prior to coming to see me. I interviewed her as I read through her form. I observed there was no light coming from her eyes. This is something I always check for. I don't feel my job is done until I see light shining from my client's eyes. It's the best yardstick I have for measuring if someone's heart and soul are smiling.

Nancy's eyes were downcast, her lips in a straight emotionless line–rather than a smile or frown. Her color seemed gray, her shoulders rolled forward, and her posture was that of a person who seemed to want to disappear, to be nonexistent.

I asked her how she was feeling.

"I'm tired all the time . . . my head always aches . . . I've lost my children to my ex-husband . . . I can't function at work anymore so I've lost my job . . . I feel like a failure at everything."

"Nancy, are you on any medication?"

It is my practice to ask all clients if they are taking any prescribed medications. I keep a reference guide to medications in my office and I look-up the side effects and read them to my clients whenever there could be questions as to how the medication might be affecting them (or if it might counteract my therapy).

It was a good thing I looked up her medications. Nancy was taking anti-seizure medication, a drug to control her hormones, and an antidepressant–simultaneously. All three medications listed liver complications as a possible side effect. I asked Nancy more questions.

"Does your body hurt right here?" I pointed to the area between her rib cage and her stomach.

"Yes–all the time."

"Do you have a slight fever, often?"

"Just about always."

"Do you have pain in your joints?"

"Yes," she said.

"Is your stool off color?"

"Yes, it's frequently light colored–how did you know?"

"Do you use alcohol often?" I asked, knowing she did as her sister had told me so.

"I've been drinking more and more often–it helps to numb out the depression."

I was in quite a predicament. I felt it likely one of the reasons my client was depressed was because she was suffering from hepatitis (an inflamed liver) and did not know it. Not being a doctor, I didn't know what I should say. The legal ramification of suggesting to a client they might have hepatitis could be vast–but on the other hand, if she kept taking her medication she might incur serious liver damage or even die.

I decided to take a risk. I told her what I suspected was possible.

"Nancy, you need to listen carefully to me now. . . look here at the PDR medication guide. Every single drug you are taking lists liver complications as a side effect. You yourself told me you have headaches, fever, joint pain, and fatigue. Those are all symptoms of possible liver trauma.

It's possible the reason you feel so down is because you are sick, not because you are depressed. If your liver isn't operating correctly it would definitely make you feel depressed."

I knew all of this because years before I suffered from a viral liver disease which I overcame with proper nutrition and by drinking water regularly.

"How long has it been since you have seen your doctor?"

"Which doctor? I go to three different doctors."

"Did three different doctors give you these medications?"

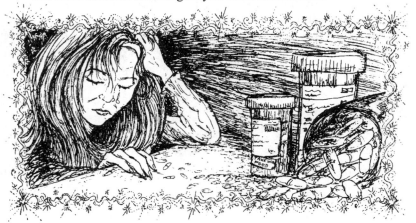

"Yes. My gynecologist gave me one medication, my psychiatrist gave me another, and my family practitioner gave me the last drug."

"How long has it been since you saw your family practitioner?"

"I guess about a year-and-a-half."

"Nancy, I don't mean to alarm you, but you need to go to your family doctor immediately and have him do blood tests. Tell him about all the medication you are on and ask him to find out if the drugs you are taking are damaging your liver. I will write your doctor a note you may take to him explaining what I am concerned about. In the meantime, keep taking your medication as it was prescribed, and get to the doctor's as fast as you can. I also want you to stop drinking alcohol immediately. Will you do these things?"

I was shaking, but I knew I had done the right thing.

"You mean I might not be crazy?"

"I don't think you are crazy at all. I know you will be fine. I will relax you, and give you suggestions that your body will heal itself rapidly, and that joy and good health will return to you immediately. Does that sound okay?"

"That sounds unbelievable," she said. "I can't remember what it is like to feel good."

"If you start believing it is possible, it will become possible," I told her. "I'm going to tape record this session for you so you can listen to it every day you feel a desire to.

There are a few other things you should start doing for yourself today—some things you can do immediately which will facilitate your wellness." I continued, "Drink at least six glasses of water a day; eat only natural healthy foods; avoid high fat foods; quit drinking alcohol and avoid coffee; and start doing some simple exercises every day—like walking or wading in a warm pool—just as much as is comfortable for you."

This advice is good advice for anyone, but in Nancy's case I believed it to be of critical importance.

"Can you do all of this for me please, and will you promise to see your doctor right away?"

"I promise. It all makes sense. I'll do it." Nancy seemed relieved.

I tranced Nancy into a pleasant state of oblivion. I suggested she feel the energy centers in her body opening, and resonating, and pulsating. I have learned these suggestions produce a state of euphoria in the client almost instantly.

I also gave Nancy all the following suggestions:

- Your body is a perfect self-healing mechanism.

- Healing energy moves through all parts of your body.

- Your body is now balancing and perfecting itself.

- Your body is ridding itself of toxins in a safe, healthy manner.

- You are turning on your own happiness.

- You are allowing your joy to surface.

- Every day you will feel better, more confident, more peaceful, and relaxed.

- There is a love and joy light shining in your heart. Each day this love and joy light will shine brighter; this love and joy light will enable you to feel happy and healthy.

- You will never again act against yourself.

- You are your own best friend, your own guardian angel.

- You keep yourself safe and happy always.

- Your creativity, strength, and courage are now surfacing.

- You only feed yourself healthy foods and positive thoughts.

- You think clearly and act in your own best interest.

- You will now act in the best interest of your family as a whole.

- You will slowly regain the trust and admiration of your children and your husband.

- You do everything with love, joy, and laughter.

- You love yourself more each day.

Before I returned her to full awareness, I suggested her subconscious would keep her energy centers open and resonating so she would always feel good, balanced, and centered. I clearly stated she was in control of herself, and could utilize self-hypnosis, as desired, to make herself feel wonderful.

When I brought Nancy back to full consciousness, I could see light in her eyes and I knew she would be okay. I said a silent prayer of thanks. I thanked her for allowing me to facilitate her wellness.

"I can't ever remember feeling this good," she said.

"You can always feel this way if you want to–in fact it was you who created this feeling inside yourself, not me. Just keep listening to this tape until you realize that you can create your own health and happiness anytime, any place, and under any circumstances."

I quickly taught Nancy simple self-hypnosis techniques and reminded her of all the things she needed to do.

"Please let me know what your doctor has to say."

As Nancy left, I finally exhaled. I felt as if I had been holding my breath for hours.

TWO WEEKS LATER

Nancy's sister called me.

"Nancy wanted me to tell you that she went to the doctor and her liver function tests were abnormal, just as you suspected," she said.

"Is her doctor furious at me for interfering with his patient?"

"No–just the opposite. He told her she looked and sounded great and she should stop taking all the medication and keep listening to the tape you made her." She went on to say, "Thanks for helping my sister. She's like a new person."

"Thanks for sending her to me and thanks for the trust you placed in me."

Gratitude danced inside my heart.

CONCLUSIONS

1. Occasionally, as a therapist, I need to go out on a limb–to take a guarded risk.

2. I feel referring someone back to his/her physician is always the smartest and safest thing to do *(and it takes the responsibility off my shoulders)*. I believe hypnotherapists should work in conjunction with physicians–not in opposition to them.

3. I always ask clients if they are on medication, because it is possible for medication to interfere with my treatment, and in some instances to depress the emotional state of the client.

4. Depression is often caused by chemicals in a person's body, poor nutrition, alcohol use, or any combination of these factors. Therefore, I always suggest that each client do the following: eat nutritious food, avoid drugs, alcohol, and other toxins, and exercise regularly. *(Regular exercise produces an increased level of endorphins in the body which is the body's own natural feel-good drug. Exercise is also a great stress reducer.)*

5. By using similar techniques to this above case study, in one year's time, four of my clients went to their physicians and obtained permission to stop taking antidepressants and/or tranquilizers. All of these clients are thriving now–they all have light in their eyes.

Connie: Part One

Overcoming Sugar Addiction
and the Stress Inherent in Being A Doctor

Connie Smith *(not her real name)* came to see me after I successfully treated her mother for depression. When she called me, the following conversation ensued:

"Ms. Griffin, this is Connie Smith. I am Shirley Talbot's daughter."

"Hello, Connie. Please call me Julie—your mom said you might be calling. How are you?"

"I'm fine, thank you, but I am hoping you can help me to get my sugar addiction under control. I'm a doctor, and I'm always telling patients to eat healthfully, so my sugar addiction makes me feel like a hypocrite."

"I'd be happy to help you, Connie. What day would be good for you?"

"May I see you Saturday morning?"

"Certainly. How about 10 a.m.?"

"Okay, I'll see you then."

THREE DAYS LATER

Connie was seated in my office as I looked through her completed intake form. She was well dressed, attractive, and clearly in her proper weight range. I spent some time asking her about her lifestyle and explaining to her how hypnosis works.

She told me how pleased she was with my treatment of her mother.

"Connie, one thing I want you to understand is that your mom got well largely because she decided it was time. In other words she chose to get well."

"Yes, but she chose to get well with you and that is why I came to see you. She was depressed for over five years; now she's not. It must have something to do with your abilities."

"All I did was give her suggestions and a feeling of choice. The real magic came from inside her. We all have magic inside us—it's just a matter of choosing to use it."

"What do you mean?"

"Everything is a choice and your ability to control your sugar intake or to change anything else about yourself depends upon your making a clear choice to change. Hypnosis will enable you to feel more inclined to do what you want to do, it will help you to unlock your own power, and your own magic–but it will *not* make you behave against your own will."

"I definitely want to control this sugar thing."

"Tell me about your sugar consumption."

"It's mostly at work when I'm stressed out."

"What stresses you at work?"

"Nurses, other doctors, patients, illness, dying, death–you name it."

"That does sound like a handful."

"I guess what bothers me the most is when someone is in pain and I can't help. I can deal with the rest of it, but that is the worst. I feel guilty about how relieved I often feel when patients die."

"I know what you mean. As I watched my mother die of cancer, I prayed for her death. It's a very difficult thing to have to do. I can help you with that during this session, too."

"How?"

"I'll give you suggestions which will put everything into proper perspective in your mind. It will be easy. Is there anything else you would like to work on?"

I always ask my clients if they would like help with any other issues because often clients will come up with a simple problem such as controlling sugar just to get into my office. Once they meet with me it is easier for them to tell me what they may have been too embarrassed to discuss on the phone.

"Actually, there is something else bothering me, but I don't know if anyone can help me with this."

"I can assist you with just about anything. Do you want to tell me what it is?"

"I can't perform oral sex on my husband. Every time I try, I choke and gag. Just the thought of it makes me sick to my stomach."

"I can help you with that, but only if you really want to do it. I don't want to give you suggestions which will enable you to do it if you don't really want to do it. Is this your idea or is your husband pressuring you?"

"Oh no, he would never pressure me. I really want to do it. I want to make him happy. I want to be able to enjoy doing it. I love making him happy and looking pretty for him. This whole thing has a negative effect on our marriage. He feels like I'm rejecting him."

"Do you know why you don't enjoy it?"

"Yes, I'm pretty sure I do. When I was 16 years old I was orally raped."

"I'm sorry."

"I think the memory of it is preventing me from enjoying oral sex now. Do you think that is possible?"

"It is very possible."

"Can you help me with this?"

"Yes, I'm sure I can. What I will do is, regress you in a safe and peaceful way, to the time the rape occurred. I will have you see it occurring as if you are watching yourself watch yourself on a movie screen. That way you will not feel like it is actually happening again."

"What is the point in my seeing it again?"

"I want you to realize that what occurred was an act of violence, not an act of sex. I want you to be able to dissociate the rape from your marriage and sex, because the rape had nothing to do with your marriage, or your husband, or sex. When you are hypnotized I will give suggestions which will enable you to helpfully reorder your feelings and emotions."

"Will it take away my feelings of guilt about what happened?"

"You feel guilty about being raped?"

"Yes. What happened was, a bunch of us were at a party and when my friends decided to leave I was offered a ride home by a guy I barely knew. When all my friends left, he said he would give me a ride home, but when we were to leave he told me he wouldn't take me home until I sucked on him. I should have just told him I would walk, but I was twenty miles away from home, and it was freezing cold and snowy. I was afraid I would freeze to death if I didn't do it."

"This guy was older than you?"

"Yes."

"And he agreed to take you home, but then put a condition on it after your friends left?"

"Yes."

"You have nothing to feel guilty about. He was older than you, he took advantage of you, and he violated you. I will help you clearly see that when you are hypnotized. When you know it with certainty, the feelings of guilt will go away."

"That will be great."

"What I want to do is deal with that issue separately from the sugar issue. Let's deal with the sugar issue today and you may come back at another time to deal with this other issue. The treatments for these two issues are entirely different. Today's session will relax you and help you move away from sugar.

I will also give you a suggestion that every time you use hypnosis you will go deeper into relaxation and it will work better than the time before. I will state that you will only accept suggestions which are truly within your own highest good. That way, if I say anything that does not feel perfect to you, your mind will simply disregard it.

Also, when you listen to the tape, its benefit will continue to increase and when you come back for your next appointment, you will have already developed an excellent ability to go into the state of hypnosis. I will give you an audio cassette to take home which will make you want to eat healthfully. You may then come back and deal with the other issue when you are ready to do so. Does that sound okay?"

"Yes, it all sounds fine."

I proceeded to explain how hypnosis works to Connie and I got her comfortably situated.

"Do you understand all I've explained to you?"

"Yes, except I am not sure about how much I should listen to the tape."

"Good question. I will be giving you one tape with two different sides. The first side has all the suggestions I give my regular weight loss clients. Even though you are not here to lose weight, you should listen to it because it contains messages suggesting that you'll prefer healthy foods. Since you are already in your ideal weight range, it will not make you lose weight because it states that you will achieve or remain at your ideal body weight. It also has motivation for exercise and positive attitude suggestions.

The other side of the tape will be a recording of this session. It will cover everything we discussed on your intake form, it will enable you to move away from sugar, and it will prepare you for our next session.

You should listen to one side of the tape each day until we meet again. I would alternate the sides from day-to-day. It is okay to miss a day, but make sure you listen to it at least five out of seven days per week. That way it will actively have the opportunity to enable you to change the way you think about food."

"What time of day should I listen to it?"

"You may listen to it anytime you want—but don't listen to it in your car. It is not safe to listen to it when you are driving because it is designed to put you into a deeply relaxed state. You may listen to it when you go to bed at night or any other time you can find 30 minutes to relax."

"What if I fall asleep when I'm listening to it? Does that mean it won't work?"

"It is perfectly fine if you fall asleep in the middle of it because hypnosis utilizes the subconscious mind and the subconscious mind is fully alert when you are asleep. Your mind pays attention to all the things it should pay attention to—even when you are sleeping."

"How is that possible?"

"Here's an example: Have you ever been sound asleep and a firetruck or an ambulance has gone by and you have slept through it?"

"Yes, I'm sure I have."

"However, I bet the sound of your baby crying three doors away wakes you up in the middle of the night every time, right?"

"Yes, that's true."

"It's because the subconscious pays attention to what it is supposed to pay attention to, *always*. As a result of this, it is fine to listen to the tape at bedtime; in fact, most of my clients say it enables them to sleep soundly."

"When will we meet next?"

"I suggest we meet about a week from now. If Saturday is a good day for you, we may have this same appointment time next week."

"Yes, I think that will be fine."

"Okay now, Connie, you may get yourself settled in. I'm going to step out for a couple of minutes but you may lie down on the couch or sit in the recliner or rocker, whichever seems most appealing. Feel free to grab a blanket or pillow and let yourself start to relax while I'm gone. I'll be right back."

When I returned to the private session room, Connie was already deeply relaxed. I proceeded to have her imagine that there was a warm wave of energy surrounding her body as she inhaled and exhaled upon my suggestion. After a few minutes of deep breathing, I had her imagine she was in Hawaii (which her intake form revealed was her favorite place) and that warm sun rays were progressively relaxing her body.

I observed the following trance indicators before I began to give therapeutic suggestions: her eyes were fluttering, her upper lip twitched occasionally, she was displaying deep belly breathing, and her body seemed to be readily accepting all the progressive relaxation suggestions as I recited them.

I then gave the following suggestions:

- You will remain calm and peaceful at work and at home.

- You will handle life's stress perfectly by eating healthfully, exercising regularly, and drinking fresh, delicious water.

- You will only feed yourself the healthiest foods and the most positive thoughts.

- Greasy, sugary, salty, and oily foods are unappealing to you; you now recognize these foods as your enemies.

- When you see junk food at work, it will be easy for you to place a visual stop sign over the food, in your mind.

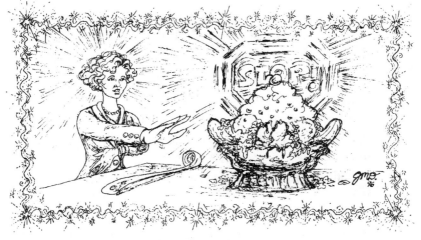

- Anytime you see sugary foods, you will be able to use your mind to picture them in black and white so they will look unappealing.

- Anytime you see sugar-filled foods you will be able to shrink them in your mind until they disappear from your vision.

- You now have complete control over the food you select.

- You now enjoy the sweet, juicy, delicious taste of fruits which are appropriate to your health.

- You now actively incorporate the appropriate amount of sweet, juicy, delicious fruit into your diet.

- Substances containing refined sugar are now unappealing to you because you have decided to be a role model of healthy eating.

- As you eat healthfully, you will feel good about yourself because you are practicing what you preach to your patients.

- As you eat healthfully, you will be setting a wonderful example for your child, your husband, and your patients.

- You will now be very conscious to eat healthfully at work, at breaks, during meals, at home, and on vacations.

- It will now be easy for you to eat healthfully because you are developing a true desire for healthy foods.

- You notice that, as you eat healthfully, you have more energy.

- You notice that, as you eat healthfully, you become emotionally stable.

- You notice that, as you eat healthfully, you become healthier.

- All the systems in your body function perfectly.

- Your body is a perfect, self-healing mechanism.

- Your blood sugar level is now balancing and perfecting itself.

- You sleep well at night, and wake happy and refreshed each day.

- You organize your grocery shopping so you do it less often.

- You select and prepare delicious healthy foods your entire family will enjoy.

- The little things that used to get on your nerves no longer affect you.

- It is easy for you to assist your patients.

- You always know the perfect thing to say to your patients to enable them to relax, feel happy, and to heal themselves.

- You are aware dying is part of living and that the soul is eternal.

- You are now able to view dying as a natural progression, as a celebration of one being returned to source.

- Inside death there is a love-filled light which heals all.

- The more trying things become at work, the more aware you are to take time to relax yourself and to eat healthfully.

- You interface well with nurses, patients, and other doctors.

- You do not allow the stress of others to affect you.

- You are able to cope appropriately with all work-related or home-based situations as they occur.

- Very soon it will be easy for you to be intimate with your husband on all levels.

- Soon you will be able to do everything you want to do.

- You are moving away from issues from the past that have prevented you from fully enjoying your marriage and your sexuality.

- Your mind, heart, and spirit are now actively healing themselves.

- Your mind is clear; your heart is full; your body heals; your soul is free; and you are happy.

- You think clearly and act in your own best interest.

- You are in complete control of your health, your happiness, and your destiny.

- Each day you will fall more in love with your family and friends, as you fall more in love with yourself.

I then gave her the following visualization suggestions:

- Visualize yourself eating healthfully.

- Visualize your family eating healthfully.

- Visualize yourself moving away from inappropriate foods and behaviors.

- Visualize yourself remaining relaxed at home and at the hospital.

- Visualize yourself taking deep relaxing breaths throughout each day.

- Visualize yourself comforting your patients.

- Visualize death as one's soul flying freely into a beautiful healing light.

- Visualize a garden in your mind that grows healthy thoughts and positive behavior.

- Visualize yourself fully enjoying your sexuality.

Next, I had her return to Hawaii in her mind and imagine that sunlight was again warming and relaxing her body. I told her that all the helpful suggestions she received during this mental vacation would continue to grow peacefully inside her.

I then had her silently affirm the following:

- I choose to eat healthfully.
- I exercise regularly and drink water often.
- I leave work issues at work and home issues at home.
- Greasy, fatty, salty, and sugary foods are no longer appealing to me.
- I eat for my health and beauty.
- I am health and beauty.
- I choose to remain relaxed at work and at home.
- I remember to take relaxation breaks and to breathe deeply several times a day.
- I stop and give thanks for all I have.
- I take time to notice how beautiful the world is.
- I am relaxed by the blueness of the sky.
- I am healed by the light of the sun.
- I am a great mother, wife, and doctor.
- I always know the perfect thing to say at the perfect time.
- I forgive myself for anything I have done wrong in the past.
- I forgive those who have wronged or injured me.
- I am now free to give and receive unconditional love and to live my life to its fullest.
- I am putting issues from the past into proper perspective so I may fully enjoy my life.
- I am allowing my sexuality to blossom and bloom.

As I returned Connie to full consciousness, I gave her a suggestion that hypnosis would work perfectly for her and she would have complete control of which suggestions she chose to accept. I also suggested that she would be able to relax more deeply and effectively each time she used hypnosis.

"How do you feel? You did great."

"I feel wonderful. That was so relaxing. My body feels really heavy, is that normal?"

"Yes, it's one of the signs you were hypnotized. Do you realize the session itself was about 30 minutes?"

"No, it felt like it was about ten minutes."

"That's because generally the deeper you go into hypnosis the shorter the time span seems. It's not always that way, but it's frequently that way."

"So that's it?"

"That's it. Just listen to your tape–one side each day; and I'll see you here this time next week."

"Is it okay if I listen to one side more than the other?"

"You should listen to each side at least once, but then you may listen to whichever side you want. Most of the time my clients prefer the side I made for them, but listen to both and see what you think."

"Okay."

"Thanks for allowing me to assist you."

RATIONALE

Since Connie needed treatment for many different issues, I decided to begin with the least threatening issues. This allowed Connie time to become comfortable with me and my techniques before we moved into less pleasant domains. During the first session I laid the ground work which would enable the second session to go smoothly:

1. I created a dynamic in which forgiveness became possible and desirable.

2. I suggested she would be able to put the past into its proper perspective.

3. I presupposed she would be able to fully enjoy her sexuality.

4. I gave suggestions which would make her feel good, powerful, and in control.

This first session not only enabled her to gain control of her eating habits, it enabled her to view herself as capable of managing all the realities in her home and work lives. When she returned for the second session she believed it would be possible for her to overcome anything.

Connie: Part Two

Ending Lingering Effects of Rape and Fostering Sexual Freedom

"Good morning, Connie. How are you?"

"I'm fine. How are you?"

"I'm very well, thank you. How did everything go this week?"

"Things went great. I listened to the tapes every day. I listened to my personalized one about twice as much as the other one."

"It's natural you would prefer the one made specifically for you."

"I did, and I believe it made me feel more relaxed at work and as a result I was able to think clearer and make better choices about food."

"So you were able to stay away from sugar?"

"Yes; actually, I don't remember even thinking about it. It just stopped being an issue."

"Wonderful. Okay then, we can move onto the next topic. Are you certain you want to proceed with this session as we discussed it last week?"

"Absolutely."

"Is there anything else you want me to know?"

"Not that I can think of."

"Okay then, I'll ask you to make yourself comfortable and I'll be back with you in a couple of minutes. You may begin to relax while I'm gone, knowing this session is going to go smoothly and peacefully."

I stepped out for a couple of minutes to allow time for the suggestion I made that the session would go smoothly to work on Connie's conscious and subconscious minds. I did my usual clearing ritual on myself, and then returned to the therapy room.

Connie seemed very relaxed when I returned to the room.

"Connie, is it okay if I lightly squeeze your wrist and tap your forehead during this session? It will help me to monitor your state."

"Sure, that will be fine."

Connie's breathing pattern and eye movements indicated to me that she had already gone into a trance.

"Okay, now I'd like you to breathe along with me for just a couple of minutes–that's right. Take in a long, slow breath . . . and exhale . . . and feel relaxed as you take in another deep breath . . . and exhale . . . and feel more peaceful as you inhale . . . and safe as you exhale . . . very good. Now with each breath you take and each sound of my voice you may continue to relax and feel even more peaceful. Also, anytime you feel me squeeze your wrist you will relax deeper and feel more peaceful. Anytime you feel me tap your forehead like this *(I made the motion)*, you will go into a safe and peaceful place in your mind and your entire body will relax. Do you understand?" Connie nodded as she went deeper.

I employed a standard progressive relaxation technique to get her to the proper depth level prior to utilizing the following therapy appropriate to her needs.

"Now, Connie, I'd like you to feel yourself being surrounded by the love and protection of the entire universe. Feel a warm, golden, glowing light surrounding you and protecting you. Allow your mind to drift and wander in the direction which is best for it to go, to help you to achieve your goals.

Feel yourself now melting into a state of absolute knowing, a state in which you can see clearly and objectively, a state where you can fine-tune your own reactions to issues from your past. That's right, feel peaceful as you notice a sense of power moving through you. Become aware you are now unlocking the power within you that will enable you to affect change in your life.

You are fully aware you will only affect the kind of changes in your thoughts and actions which are appropriate to your highest good. You are also aware this entire process will be peaceful and will enable you to feel free to fully express your own sexual desires.

Drift deeper now *(I began a process where I lightly squeezed her wrist approximately every 20 seconds, so she would continually go deeper)* as you sense a feeling of euphoria filling your physical body and as you silently speak this prayer of protection along with me now:

- We ask Connie's higher power to protect us as Connie explores her past and makes helpful changes in her mindset. Please keep us safe today and always. Thank you for your love. Thank you for your guidance. Thank you.

Now Connie, you may speak inside yourself this prayer of forgiveness:

- I forgive myself for anything I have done wrong in the past. I forgive anyone who has wronged or injured me. I am now free to give and receive unconditional love and experience joy to its fullest on this and all the days of my life."

Connie's body was very still. I could barely tell she was breathing. She had a serene look about her which told me the process was going to be simple.

"Connie, as I count from one to five you may allow yourself to travel backwards in time to the incident which is currently preventing you from enjoying your sexuality to its fullest. At the count of five it will be as if you are watching yourself watch yourself on a movie screen. You will be able to view the incident in a totally objective way, as an outsider would view it. Your body and mind will remain calm and peaceful throughout this experience."

I squeezed Connie's wrist a couple more times before I began the count.

"One, see and feel yourself going back in time through the glowing, love-filled light of the universe; two, feel yourself becoming stronger and happier; three, remain warm and relaxed; four, almost there, relaxed and peaceful; and five, now safely seeing the past as if you are watching yourself watch yourself in a movie."

As I said 'five' I could see Connie's eyes moving rapidly under her closed eyelids. I assumed she was visually recreating the past.

"Connie, tell me where you are."

"I'm in Grafton."

"How old are you?"

"I'm 15."

"What's going on?"

"I'm with Ron."

"What is happening?"

"We are in his car and we are leaving the party. He's supposed to take me home."

"Are you going home?"

"No, he's stopping the car. He's telling me he won't take me home unless I let him put his dick in my mouth."

"Do you want to do it?"

"No, it scares me and I don't like him."

"What do you say to him?"

"I won't do it."

"Does he take you home then?"

"No, he just starts unzipping his pants and taking it out."

Connie continued to tell the story in a very detached way. I was pleased at how calm she remained. I continued to squeeze her wrist each time I asked her a question.

"Now what is happening?"

"I'm looking the other way. I don't want to see it."

"What does he do next?"

"He tells me I can be like that, but we aren't going anywhere until I put it in my mouth."

"Connie, please see clearly the position you were in. You were far away from home, and you were with someone who was trying to make you do something against your will. Is that correct?"

"Yes."

"What happened next?"

"He shut off the car and the heater. I was crying and getting cold. Watching it now I think it went on for about ten minutes although I remember when it was actually happening to me it felt like an hour. I eventually did what he asked because I was terrified and I wanted to go home."

"How did you feel about this man?"

"I felt like he was terrible and that he might hurt me."

"Can you see you acted in a way to protect yourself?"

"Yes."

"Can you see you were victimized by someone who was older than you and stronger than you?"

"Yes."

"Can you see very clearly this man who victimized you is not your husband?"

"Yes."

"Can you now become aware that what occurred in this picture was not sex, but rather violence?"

"Yes."

"Will you now be able to separate this incident from any sexual practices you decide to enjoy in the future?"

"Yes."

"I'd like you to do some things in your mind which will help you to clarify that love and sex have nothing to do with coercion, violence, or rape, okay?"

"Yes."

"I'd like you to imagine you have a big bucket of paint and you are writing the word rapist over the part of the picture Ron is in. Can you do that?"

"Yes."

"What color is the paint?"

"It's red."

"Good."

"Now, I'd like you to take more paint and write the word violence over the part of the picture where you are being victimized. Okay?"

"Yes."

"What color is that paint?"

"It's black."

"Very good."

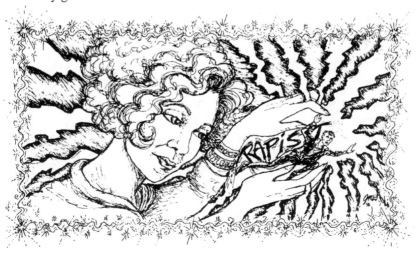

"Now, I'd like you to see in your mind this picture of the past getting smaller and smaller and changing from full color into black and white. As this picture becomes smaller and smaller, I would like you to picture yourself becoming stronger and more powerful. As you become stronger and more powerful, I would like you to feel yourself breaking through a barrier which has prevented you from fully enjoying sex. You are very strong now and you can do anything you want to do.

I'd like you to notice now that the picture is very tiny, in fact, you can barely see it. It is just a faint, distant memory, too small to affect you, too tiny to interfere with your happiness. Perhaps it might even disappear. It's your choice. You can make it disappear and never think of it again, or you can choose to remember you had the experience, survived the experience, and are now stronger because of the experience."

"I'm going to keep it tiny."

"That's good; it proves that you are strong."

"Now, it's time to have some fun. Are you ready?"

"Yes."

"Good, now I'd like you to travel back through a warm white light into your current reality, remaining deeply relaxed as I count from one to five." *(I recited the count)*

"I'd like you to see another movie screen. I'd like you to see a very sexy image of your husband on the screen. That's right; see him looking his most handsome and desirable."

There was a smile on Connie's face.

"Now, I'd like you to paint the word lover next to your husband's image on the screen. *(I paused)* What color is the paint?"

"It's pink."

"Good."

"Now, picture yourself on the screen with him, in his arms, and paint the word 'love' next to the two of you. *(I paused)* What color is the paint?"

"It's pink."

"Now I'd like you to picture yourself kissing his mouth, his face, his neck, his fingers. Now see yourself sucking on his fingers and notice how good it feels to have his fingers in your mouth. Notice how warm and soft your mouth feels and how relaxed your jaw and throat are when you suck on his fingers."

Connie's body language told me she was comfortable in all she was imagining.

"Now, Connie, I would like you to become aware of the fact that your mouth, jaw, and throat will remain this relaxed when you decide to take your husband's penis in your mouth. In fact you can actively be the initiator. You may decide you want it in your mouth and you can reach out and take it and put it in your mouth.

Or you may imagine you are enjoying the sensation of taking his penis into your mouth little by little. You may notice how beautiful it is and you may enjoy the mixed feelings of comfort and sexuality you experience when you suck on it.

It is okay to imagine this scene anyway you want to imagine it. Allow yourself to picture it in your mind, to feel the love you feel toward your husband, and to feel the desire you feel for him. You may allow a feeling of warm passion to grow inside your heart and pelvic region when you picture this."

I could see by her expressions and body language Connie was enjoying the scenes she was creating in her mind.

"As you continue picturing this in your mind, you may become aware that very soon you will be able to create it as your reality. That's right, you are aware of the following:

- You are passion.
- You are free to fulfill your desires.
- You are free to fulfill your husband's desires.
- Your mouth, throat, and belly will remain appropriately relaxed when you participate in sexual activities.
- You will look very beautiful to your husband with his penis in your mouth.
- You can use your imagination to help you to fantasize about all you want to fulfill sexually.
- When the time is perfect, you will be able to act out your fantasies.
- All you and your husband want to share together is right and good.
- You are passion.
- You are love.
- Your love and passion will continue to blossom and bloom."

I then returned Connie to full conscious awakening. As she became alert, she was smiling and laughing.

"That was so much fun."

"All of it?"

"I meant the last few minutes, but the part where I was writing on the screen and shrinking Ron was almost as much fun."

"I have this session on tape, but I think you should probably only listen to the sexy parts of you and your husband enjoying each other. I will erase it up until that point, and give you the rest. There is no point in your hearing the other parts again."

"I'd like to have the whole thing, Julie. I will mostly listen to the sexy part, but I think I want to hear the part where I shrank Ron again. Is that okay?"

"Just so long as you don't live in the past. It's time for you to move into feelings of love and passion—not to dwell on the past."

"I will, I promise."

I knew she would.

Horsing Around In Her Head
A Woman, Her Horse & Self-Hypnosis

Throughout 1994, I was a regular on Massachusetts' Continental Cable's, *Healthy Mind and Body Show*. The show's host, Robin Reale Allen, complained to me one day that everyone at her riding club made fun of her riding and her horse's ill-bred nature.

"I can't believe it. They told me I shouldn't even enter the competition. They said I haven't been riding long enough and Shawnee doesn't fit in with their horses. They really hurt my feelings; what a bunch of snobs," Robin said, one evening at J.C. Hillary's Restaurant, where we ate dinner after every show.

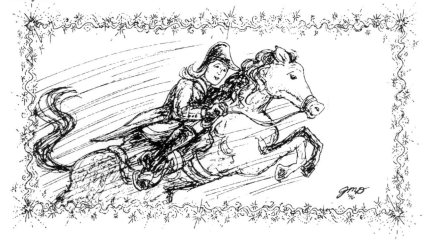

"Robin, why don't you allow me to hypnotize you so that you will be able to ride to the best of your ability?"

"Thanks, Julie, but I'm still afraid of being hypnotized. Part of me really wants to be hypnotized, but part of me is afraid. I hope that doesn't hurt your feelings."

"Of course it doesn't hurt my feelings. You know what though?"

"What?"

"I can still help you do your best at the competition."

"How?"

"I can teach you how to hypnotize yourself–that way you will be in control of the whole thing and you won't be afraid."

"Do you really think I can do it myself?"

"I know you can. In fact, people hypnotize themselves all the time accidentally."

"What do you mean?"

"Have you ever said to yourself, 'I know I'm going to get the cold that's going around' and then whammo, you catch it?"

"Sure, hasn't everyone?"

"Have you ever said to yourself, 'I don't have time to get sick right now, I'm not going to catch the cold that's going around' and then you remained healthy?"

"Yes, I have done that, too."

"Or, have you ever had an important question in your mind or a decision to make and have said to someone, 'Let me sleep on that,' and then woke-up the next day with the best answer to the question?"

"I've done that many times."

"Those are all forms of self-hypnosis. Self-hypnosis occurs anytime you give your subconscious a direct suggestion. The suggestions are accepted in the deepest way when you are either highly focused or relaxed, but it often works even without a focused or relaxed state.

Other times you have hypnotized yourself would include: when you drive your car and you realize you don't remember driving part of the trip, or, when you watch a movie and you get so caught up in the movie you actually jump when someone on the screen throws a punch, or, anytime you read a good book and you become so engrossed in the book you feel like you can't put the book down. These are all forms of hypnosis."

"All of the things you are describing happen to me."

"That means you will be a good candidate for self-hypnosis."

"How do I do it?"

"You can do it any place or anytime, but I think it will be easiest for you to do it at home when you are going to sleep at night. All you need to do is to close your eyes, take in a few long, slow, deep breaths, and picture yourself doing well at the competition. I suggest you imagine the following things once you get into bed at night:

- ◆ Picture and feel yourself and Shawnee totally connected mentally–operating synchronously with one another.

- Imagine you are drawing into yourself from the universal energy field, the essence of perfect riding abilities.

- Picture yourself and Shawnee completing all the jumps perfectly.

- Imagine Shawnee behaving like a championship horse.

- Imagine yourself riding Shawnee to a gas station that has pumps containing the bloodline of all the greatest champion horses. Imagine yourself infusing Shawnee with this blood.

- Picture yourself becoming increasingly confident about your abilities as an equestrian.

- Hear the sound of everyone congratulating you after the event.

- Picture the look on everyone's faces when you do extremely well in competition.

- Imagine how great you feel when you prove how good you and Shawnee actually are."

"That's all I have to do?"

"Yes."

"How many times do I do it?"

"You can do it as often as you want but the more you do it the better it will work. When is the show?"

"It's next weekend."

"I suggest you do it every night until the show. That way, your mind will have the opportunity to accept the suggestions as its new truth."

"That sounds easy enough. But what if I don't come out of hypnosis?"

"You don't have to worry about that. You will automatically come out of it if you want to, but I suggest you do it in bed and give yourself a suggestion that it is okay to fall asleep afterwards. This will help you to sleep at night because you will feel very relaxed as you do it."

"Can I give myself other suggestions, too?"

"Of course you can. You can use this for anything you want. In fact you don't have to be in bed to do it. You can do it anywhere simply by doing the following:

- take a few deep breaths;

- tell your body to relax;

- focus your mind; and

- give yourself the desired suggestions.

You can do a long process where you go deeply into a focused or relaxed state, or you may do it in seconds. The more you practice, the faster you will be able to go into the state. The important thing to remember is, you will come out of it precisely when you want to. That way you won't be afraid to do it."

"That sounds too good to be true."

"I promise you it's true and it works. I've never told you this before, but I do the entire television show with you while I'm in a trance."

"You do? Why?"

"Because it stops me from being nervous, and it helps me to speak articulately and to remember what I want to say."

"Is that why you are so smooth on the air?"

"Yes, I'd be a wreck otherwise. I have given myself what are called post-hypnotic suggestions. A post-hypnotic suggestion is a suggestion that goes into affect after the hypnosis session is actually over."

"How do you do that?"

"I gave myself a suggestion that anytime I get to the television station I will automatically enter into a deeply relaxed and highly focused state which enables me to perform perfectly."

"I could do that with the horse show?"

"Certainly. You may give yourself these post-hypnotic suggestions:

♦ the closer it gets to the day of the show the more confident you become;

♦ at the show, you and Shawnee will both be relaxed, focused, and confident, and you will both perform magnificently."

"I like this! Do you think I can actually do it?"

"Anyone can do it. I wish everyone would use self-hypnosis because it makes everything so much easier. I use it for long-distance swimming, and all kinds of other things."

"That's amazing–no wonder you get so much done."

As Robin and I ate our dinner, and gossiped about mutual friends, we paused to plan for our next show together.

"I have an idea; why don't you teach self-hypnosis on the next program? Can you do that?"

"Sure, I'd love to teach hypnosis on the air."

We proceeded to pick my next on-air date which was three weeks later.

THREE WEEKS LATER

I arrived at the television station a few minutes early and watched Robin conclude her interview with a man who had just traveled, to and hiked into, the mountains of Peru. I was scheduled to go on after the commercial break.

During the break, the stage hands quickly moved me onto the set and wired a microphone through the sleeve of my dress and up onto my lapel. The explorer remained on the set with us. As the camera person gave us the five second countdown cue, I felt myself becoming increasingly focused and ready.

"Welcome back, everyone. Joining us is hypnotist, Julie Griffin, director of the Hypnotherapy Training Company. Julie is going to teach us how to hypnotize ourselves. Good evening, Julie. Thank you for being here."

"You are welcome, Robin; it's always an honor and pleasure to be here. Thank you for the warm welcome."

I explained on live television how hypnosis works and how viewers could hypnotize themselves. Part way through my instructions, the fellow who had traveled to Peru spoke to me.

"Julie, how could I use self-hypnosis when I am traveling?"

"That's a great question. You could use it any number of ways. Here are a few suggestions you can give to yourself:

♦ It is now easy for me to study and learn foreign languages.

♦ It is now easy for me to understand foreign cultures.

♦ My body clock and systems adjust themselves perfectly in foreign cultures and time zones.

♦ I am one with the universe; therefore I am comfortable, peaceful, and healthy wherever I am.

♦ My body adjusts itself perfectly when I eat foreign foods and live in foreign climates.

♦ My body adjusts itself perfectly in varying altitudes.

♦ I prepare my body for hiking by training properly.

♦ I train properly by exercising regularly, eating healthfully, and drinking fresh purified water.

These are the type of suggestions I would give to myself if I were you. I think they will create the perfect mindset for what you do."

"So do I. That really sounds helpful, thank you," he said.

I remembered Robin's horse competition had come and gone.

"Robin, I must ask you, how did you do at the horse show?"

Robin had a big smile on her face. She proceeded to tell the viewing audience about how I taught her self-hypnosis.

"All I did was relax myself and give myself the type of suggestions Julie mentioned. It was very easy," Robin said.

"How did you do at the event?"

"We won the blue ribbon. Everyone was amazed, including me, but Shawnee and I won the blue ribbon. It was one of the best days of my life. I was just hoping not to be embarrassed, but we actually won first place! Thank you for helping me."

"You did it all yourself. I'm proud of you."

I then addressed my television audience directly. "So there it is folks, proof we can all affect the outcomes of what we do, using the power of our own minds."

A Not So Merry Christmas

Post-Traumatic Stress Syndrome & Agoraphobia –
Hypnotist Heal Thyself

It was 6:40 a.m. on Christmas eve morning, 1994. I was on my way into my office to work with a client who had begged me to fit him in before I left for my family holiday. A nor'easter was in the air, causing an intense blustering rainstorm. There were tree limbs down everywhere. It was all I could do to keep my umbrella from blowing inside out in the storm.

As I attempted to steady my umbrella, a man tore out of the alley and charged at me like a wild animal. He let out one long, sinister sounding karate yelp before he knocked me to the ground.

I didn't know what was happening; it occurred so quickly. Was I about to be killed, robbed, or raped? I didn't know. All I knew was some maniac was punching me ferociously. I felt like I was in the middle of a nightmare. No one was around to help me, and at the time I was in shock and unable to help myself.

Although I am usually street-wise, the storm distracted me from my normal state of readiness, making me a prime candidate to be victimized. After an extended struggle, the man grabbed my bag and ran.

As the man ran away, I felt a great sense of relief because his departure with my bag indicated his purpose had been to rob me–not to kill me or rape me. My sense of relief disappeared in less than two minutes, when the man realized he had run away with a bag other than my purse. Suddenly, he charged at me again. To my horror, he knocked me down and beat me again, but this time I knew what was happening, so I responded in a way as to protect myself.

I screamed as loudly as I could, in hopes of drawing attention to myself. With my free hand I threw my purse away from myself so he would have to get away from my body in order to get what he really wanted–my money. I screamed as he beat me and as he yelled, "Give me your fucking money–bitch".

I shrieked, "It's over there, I threw it away."

Finally, he stopped hitting me, grabbed my purse, and ran away–this time for good. I didn't know what to do. At first I believed the robber had my keys and that I wouldn't be able to get into my office or my apartment. After a few minutes, I remembered the keys were in my hand when I was

126

attacked. I searched the ground in the dark for them. In several minutes time, I found my keys, along with the first bag the predator stole.

I decided to go directly to my office and call the police because it was close by and I was supposed to meet my client. It was still pouring and my umbrella had been destroyed in the attack. By the time I got to my office I looked like a drowned rat. My coat was mud-caked, my hair was dripping wet, and my make-up was running down my face.

When I got to my office, my client was not there. I called the police. A sympathetic policewoman took down my recollection of the incident.

"Miss, shall I send a cruiser out to assist you? Do you need an ambulance?"

"No, thanks. There is no point to anyone coming now. It's over, I'm safe now." I said, trying to convince myself.

"Were you physically injured?"

"He beat me, but I'm not bleeding and nothing is broken."

As she instructed me on how to cancel my credit cards and bank accounts, I kept breaking down in hysterics.

"I'm sorry, officer. I just can't fight the urge to cry anymore."

"It's okay. It's perfectly understandable. Are you sure you don't want to see a police officer?"

"No. I just want to go home, bathe, and straighten out all this business. I need to go home for Christmas in a couple of hours. Oh my God, that bastard stole my bus ticket."

"Do you need emergency cash, Miss?"

"No, I have friends I can call. This just sucks–all this horror over $2.00 and a bus ticket to Durham, NH."

"I'm glad that's all he got and I'm glad you are okay. This is very strange because I had a premonition about it while I was driving to work."

"A premonition? What do you mean?"

"It was about the weather. I had a thought that a woman outside alone in the dark, in this weather, under an umbrella, would be a sitting duck."

"I certainly was. All I can say is, that idiot bought himself a lot of bad karma for $2.00."

"He sure did. I hope you can figure out a way to have a Merry Christmas in spite of him–and, Miss, call us back if you need to–even if you just need to talk."

I sat in my office until I realized it was 7:20 and that my 7:00 appointment had not shown-up. I had an appointment with an alcoholic who claimed he wanted to quit drinking. I extended myself to see him at a time when I normally would have been home sleeping. I was viciously attacked for nothing because the client never showed-up. I felt violated by the mugger and by my client.

I made my way home, looking over my shoulder the entire way. It was now daylight, but I was still terrified. At home, I quickly locked the door behind me, walked into my apartment, and collapsed. I took off my muddied coat and wrapped myself up in an old quilt I inherited from my mother. I grabbed the phone and called my sister.

"Abby. It's me. I need help."

"Oh my God, what's the matter?"

"I was just attacked and robbed. I'm safe now, but the jerk took all my money and credit cards. He even stole my bus ticket."

"I'm coming to get you right now," Abby said.

"There is no hurry. It will take me an hour to cancel my credit cards and bank accounts, and to pack. You may get here at your leisure because it will take me a while to pull things together."

"I'm leaving right now."

As I hung-up the phone and cried hysterically again, I realized for the first time that I was physically injured. I had screamed so loud I injured my vocal chords. It felt like I had strep throat and my shoulders felt like they had been ripped-out of their sockets.

As I took off my wet clothes and got in the shower, I realized my arms were both bruised. This realization caused me to become more hysterical. I got in and out of the shower as quickly as I could, because I didn't want to look at the bruises. I dressed and phoned the appropriate agencies to cancel my credit cards and bank accounts.

It was very difficult to talk because my throat was hurting more each moment. Every time I talked to a different credit card agency and told the story of the attack, I became more upset.

In an hour's time, my sister was there, holding me and comforting me. We quickly packed and got out of town as fast as we could. During the one hour ride to New Hampshire, I had recurrent anxiety attacks.

"Abby, I can't see your kids in this condition. They won't understand why I can't control my emotions."

"It will be okay. After I talked to you, the kids heard me crying and asked me what was wrong. I decided to tell them the truth. I told them a bad man hurt you, but I was going to get you and that you would be okay. I told them I was crying because I was sad that you are sad."

"Did they understand what you were saying?"

"It was really amazing. It was just like you taught us at our parents' meeting."

"What do you mean?"

"You said that when you tell a child the truth about a situation, the child will automatically develop healthy coping mechanisms to whatever is going on—that it is only when you hide things from them or lie that they act out inappropriately. It's true. I told the kids the truth and they handled it fine. Besides, it is good for them to know there are maggots out there. It might protect them in the future."

When we got to Abby's, the kids showered me with affection. I was able to keep my emotions under control by putting myself in a light trance.

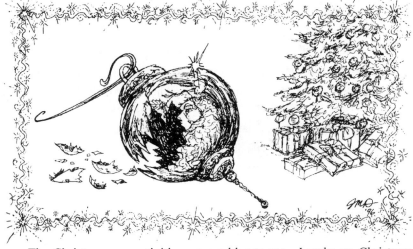

The Christmas eve activities were a blur to me. I woke-up Christmas morning in a lot of pain. My throat was on fire, my back hurt, and both my hips ached. When I got in the shower, I saw bruises on my shoulders which looked like fingerprints, and large black-and-blue marks on my hips. Seeing the bruises upset me again, but I put myself in trance so I wouldn't continually become hysterical.

I quickly got dressed and joined my family. I tried to act like I was okay, but, while my family opened gifts, I fantasized about inflicting grave bodily injury upon my assailant. I pictured myself getting a gun, shooting him, stabbing him with a knife, and cutting off his testicles. Throughout Christmas day, I thought of little other than hurting the person who stole my feeling of safety.

I vowed when I returned to Boston I would behave in the same way as I behaved before the attack. I told myself that what happened was just a random occurrence–that the terrible man was no longer out there and that I could walk the streets without fear. I did not want to allow the incident to affect my way of being any more than it already had.

When I returned to my apartment, I felt safe and sound until a policeman telephoned.

"Hello, Ms. Griffin?"

"Yes?"

"This is Detective Good Cop *(not his real name)* from the Boston PD. I've been assigned to your case."

"My case?"

"Yes. We are still trying to find the man who robbed you. But I need some more details of the incident from you."

All of a sudden the entire event was back in my face. I became emotional as I described the scene.

"I'm sorry, officer. I thought I was over this."

"It's okay, Miss. In fact, most people who are assaulted need to see a psychologist to get over it. Do you have someone you can talk to?"

"Yes, I said. I'll see to that."

"Miss, I need to warn you about a few things."

"You need to warn me?"

"Yes. You said you had a checkbook in your purse?"

"Yes."

"What about keys to your apartment?"

"No. I had the keys in my hand."

"Good."

"It is unlikely he would burglarize your apartment, but what may happen in cases like this is that the mugger gets a female accomplice to call the victim about a week after the mugging."

"Why?"

"The accomplice claims she found your purse and wants to come over and give it to you. Then they come over and rob you again. In cases like this, they have even forcibly taken the victim to an ATM machine and made him take out all his cash. They always wait about a week after the initial robbery to allow time for the victim to get his bank cards replaced."

"Oh, my God. I thought the horror was over."

"I don't mean to scare you, but it is my job to warn you. It probably will not happen, but if anyone calls claiming to have your purse, tell them to bring it to Police District 4 and that you will pick it up there. That way, if it's a real call, you will get your purse, and, if it's a ruse, you won't be hurt again."

"Thank you for warning me. I know I would have fallen for that."

"A lot of people have fallen for that."

"Do you live alone, Miss?"

"Yes."

"In the future, when you leave your apartment, you should always leave the radio on next to the door so it sounds like someone is home. It is even better if you leave your television turned-on to a talk show, because it will sound like there is more than one person in your apartment. Usually, if it sounds like someone is home, they will go away. You should also be careful going into and out of the hallways of your building. Make sure everything is well lit. Don't walk into dark entryways."

"Officer, do you think you will find this guy?"

"Honestly, I doubt it. We believe he robbed six different women the same day he robbed you. He must have been desperate. I'll let you know if we nab him."

"Thanks for all your help."

As I hung-up the phone, I felt afraid again, but for the first time in my life I actually liked the police. I told myself I would heed all the advice Detective Good Cop gave me, but I was still going to resume my normal life.

I was proud of the way I jumped back into life. I had been coming and going as I pleased and was planning a New Year's eve party when the phone rang.

"Julie, it's Mel." It was my buddy, Melanie.

"I was just mugged. I think it was the same guy who robbed you." She went on to describe the man who robbed her. The description matched the man who assaulted me.

"Oh, my God, are you okay?"

"Yes, I threw my purse as soon as he came at me, because I remembered you said that stopped him from beating you."

"What did he do?"

"He ran after the purse, picked it up, and kept running."

"He didn't hurt you?"

"No, but I had over $300.00 in my purse and it's all gone."

"Oh, I'm sorry–but I'm glad he didn't hit you. I would gladly give $300.00 to not have these bruises on my body."

"I'm really shaken. It took a while for the cops to come because they were all in Brookline."

"Why were they all in Brookline?"

"Don't you know what happened in Brookline?"

"No."

"Some maniac right-to-lifer shot up two abortion clinics. A lot of people were shot and at least two women were killed."

I felt myself snap inside. It was too much to hear. It was too much dark truth to know in such a short space of time. Melanie's robbery made me realize that evil was still lurking in alleys, preying on people like me. Far worse, some maniac with a gun, was killing people in my own backyard, in the name of Christ.

I offered to pick up Melanie by cab, and to bring her back to my place.

"No, I need to stay here in my own apartment. Thanks, but I need to be here. My parents are on their way over to bring me some money. I'll be okay."

"I'm glad you have your parents. Call me if you need anything."

"You do the same."

I had nightmares all night about being robbed and raped. I woke-up at 4:00 a.m. after only five hours of sleep. I couldn't get back to sleep. I watched infomercials until dawn. At dawn, I decided to go to the health club, but when I got dressed, I felt paralyzed to leave my apartment.

I found myself writing at my computer and the next thing I knew it was 6:00 p.m. I had talked myself out of leaving the apartment all day.

I went to bed around 11:00 p.m. but woke-up again at 4:00 a.m. to the same variety of nightmares. I read a book until I fell asleep, but the nightmares returned.

The same thing went on for two more days. I realized I had not left my apartment for four days.

Finally, it was Thursday and I had a medical appointment I could not miss. My gynecologist's office was just doors away from where one of the abortion clinic murders had occurred, just days before. By the time I got to see my doctor, Jacqueline Starer, I was completely over-wrought. I told her about the mugging and confessed I hadn't left my apartment in over four days.

"Julie, you need to see a psychologist. You might be developing agoraphobia."

"I know I'm sick, but going outside is just too difficult. I'm amazed I made it here. My whole body hurts from stress. I haven't been sleeping."

"It sounds like post-traumatic stress syndrome. Julie, you need to go outside every day so you don't develop full-blown agoraphobia. I'm going to prescribe some tranquilizers. You may take one of these up to three times a day. These will relax you enough so you will be able to leave your apartment and so you can sleep at night. Try to maintain a normal schedule and see a psychologist as soon as you can."

"Okay, I'll do it."

I left Dr. Starer's office and walked across the street to a pharmacy and filled the prescription. As soon as the pharmacist handed me the pills, I opened the bottle, and popped one into my mouth.

I walked into a coffee shop and sat down, hoping the tranquilizer would quickly take affect. About two cups of coffee and a pastry later, I felt a warm feeling inside myself which told me the pill was working. It still wasn't easy, but I went outside and waited for the train to take me home. I stopped to buy groceries but got myself home as quickly as I could.

That night, I took another tranquilizer, hoping it would enable me to sleep through the night. It didn't. I only managed to sleep for about five hours and bad dreams plagued me.

There was one thought which kept running through my mind since the attack, that thought was: *what if I had died without having written my book?* I had been thinking of writing a book of hypnotherapy scripts. It seemed queer to me at the time that this was the most prevalent thought on my mind.

It seemed as though I should have been thinking: *what if I had died without ever having seen my loved ones or friends again?* Or perhaps, *what if I had died without ever having a baby?* Yet those thoughts were not on my mind. The overwhelming question in my mind continued to be, *what if I had died without having written my book?*

So I began compiling every hypnotherapy script I had ever written. I searched my closets, my notebooks, my case files, and I came up with a multitude of disjointed, half-written scripts. One by one, I entered the scripts into my computer. As I typed them, I established a consistent format which would unite them as integral parts of the same work.

I would get up in the morning and start writing, editing, and rewriting. I had food delivered to my home when I was too frightened to go out.

I took the prescribed tranquilizers only if I had to go out or at bedtime. I didn't want to become dependent upon pills and I didn't want them to make me feel lethargic to a point where I would not be able to write.

I tried to convince myself to see a psychologist, but the only one I trusted was far away and I was still too terrified to travel far–even when I medicated myself.

The tranquilizers enabled me to go to the grocery store and post office. There was a shopping plaza only three blocks from my apartment and, under the influence of the tranquilizers, I was able to go to it in broad daylight.

I still could not go out early in the morning or after dark–but I discovered that if I took a tranquilizer 30 minutes before I went outside, I would feel only slight physical discomfort. I found I was still unwilling to force myself to go outside every day, but, every second or third day I would make myself go out for food and necessities. The rest of the time I would distract myself from my bizarre behavior by working on the book.

The book made me feel powerful and it gave me back a sense of purpose. I would immerse myself in the book for hours at a time. The book was like a life-raft which kept me mentally afloat.

One day, I realized I could not stand looking at the walls of my apartment any more. I had spent too much time looking at the same walls. Had I been in a normal state of mind, I would have rented a car and left town–or simply gone for a walk. But those thoughts did not enter my mind. Instead, I reached inside of one of my closets and pulled out my artists' paints.

Suddenly, I found myself painting my bedroom walls in vibrant colors. First, it was just random colorful shapes of red, pink, blue, and gold–but after a period of time, I realized I was actually painting a mural. Next, I painted the doors to match, and then the light switches. It seemed as though I was trying to paint my way out of the dark place I had landed in inside my mind. I painted until I ran out of paint and then I started writing again.

I continued on this way for weeks until the time came that I had scheduled a day class in hypnotherapy. I had an outside faculty member coming in to teach metaphysical hypnosis with me. I did not want to teach under the influence of tranquilizers so I managed to get to my office in a drug-free state. It was only a five block walk, but by the time I arrived at the classroom my entire body ached from stress. It occurred to me that this is how people suffering from post-traumatic stress syndrome feel every day.

My metaphysics teacher, Kendra Bond, knew of the trauma I was experiencing. She offered to use me as a subject in her teaching.

"Julie, what is the biggest conflict you are experiencing as a result of the attack?"

"It's hard to say, but I guess the worst thing is that I feel like the universe let me down. I used to believe that, because I am a good person doing good work, the universe would always protect me. But, it seems to me now, the universe turned its back on me when I most needed protection."

"Julie, do you understand that we draw into ourselves everything that occurs in our lives?"

"Yes—at least, I thought I did. But, Kendra, I would not have called this into myself."

"It's probably a karmic balance coming into play from something in a former life."

"Kendra, I don't mean to seem rude or to discount the theory entirely but sometimes isn't a banana just a banana? Isn't it possible I was just in the wrong place at the wrong time?"

"A banana is never just a banana. We need to find out why your subconscious allowed the attack to occur. Then we need to release the attack and its ramifications from your soul so you can let go of all the negative energy pertaining to it which you are carrying inside you."

"That sounds reasonable on the surface, but I am too afraid to go under and deal with the attack. I can't stand the thought of trancing into the scene, I keep doing it in my dreams—I'm not going to do it on purpose, even in the name of therapy."

"We can use a remote." Kendra suggested.

"A remote?"

"Yes. I can put someone else into trance and ask that your Wise One speak through the remote and tell us why the attack took place."

"I don't want to put anyone else through such an experience."

"It won't harm the remote. The remote will experience the knowledge in a disinterested way. I do this type of work all the time. Debra, will you serve as a remote for this?"

A student in the class, Debra Daly, stood-up, walked closer to us, and said, "Sure, I'd be happy to."

Kendra put Debra into a deep trance, while I sat watching. Once Debra was hypnotized, Kendra asked that Debra call forth the *Wise One* of me to speak through her to give information which would assist me.

After a time, my Wise One started speaking through Debra and giving the following information:

- Julie is greatly loved by the universe.

- She was not betrayed by the universe. The universe allowed the attack to occur to prevent greater harm from occurring.

Kendra asked, "Wise One, how can this be so?"

- Julie was on a course that would have caused her far greater harm emotionally and physically. The attack was necessary to stop her from proceeding on the course she was on. It is unfortunate such a dramatic occurrence was necessary, but it was the only way.

- Julie needs to become mindful that, even when things seem to be going wrong, we are always protecting her and directing her toward her highest good. When she fully regains this knowledge, she will be healed from negative lingering thoughts which are currently wrecking havoc inside her energy system.

Kendra asked, "Are there any other things we need to correct or be aware of?"

- Yes. This incident has greatly fragmented Julie's soul. Her beliefs and concepts have been shattered. She needs to be whole again.

Kendra asked, "Wise One, how do I facilitate Julie's wholeness?"

- You already know how. Trust and use your knowledge.

Kendra thanked the Wise One for its assistance and thanked the universe for its continued protection. She then brought Debra (the remote subject) back to full conscious awakening and thanked her for her participation.

As she returned to full consciousness, it was obvious Debra was having an abreaction to the information which had come through her. She said, "I feel sick to my stomach."

Kendra placed Debra back into trance and had her disconnect herself from the lingering energy and its negative effects. Kendra gave Debra several suggestions designed to create a healthy balance inside her. She also called for a team of spirit healers to facilitate Debra's energy system coming into balance.

I was upset that Debra incurred a negative physical reaction as a result of helping me. I openly questioned Kendra about the validity of assisting one person at the risk of another.

"Debra had this response because it reminded her subconscious of a similar event which occurred in her own history. Her past caused the reaction–not yours," Kendra explained.

"But this memory would not have been triggered and she would not have had this response had she not been involved in my process. I feel like I harmed her by allowing her to assist me."

"That's not true. It is the negative energy of her own memories which caused the reaction. The negative energy will continue to harm her if we do not release it. We can release it in the same manner as we released negative energy from you. I will do that now and it will free her from similar responses in the future," Kendra said.

"I still don't like it."

"If we hadn't used her as a remote, we would not be aware she has issues that need to be released. Don't you see, none of this was random? It is all occurring in divine order."

"I respect that in theory, but right now, all I can see is Debra feeling sick because she helped me."

"You may allow that thought to leave your mind so you will be able to view this as a positive process."

"I'll try."

"Don't try, just do it!" Kendra commanded.

Kendra finished doing her work on Debra and then she told me she had work she needed to do on me directly.

"Don't worry. This is easy work. Just make yourself comfortable and go into a relaxed state."

I followed Kendra's instructions and put myself in a deep trance.

Kendra then made the following suggestions:

- you may now begin to reconnect all parts of yourself;

- feel yourself connecting golden cords to all parts of you that were previously fragmented;

- feel yourself actively drawing all your parts back together;

- feel yourself becoming whole again as you imagine you are sewing yourself back together with wonderful golden cords;

- feel healing wings of angels soothing and comforting you;

- your body, mind, and spirit are becoming whole again;

- you may now let go of any negative effects of anything that has occurred in your life, particularly the events pertaining to this session;

- allow your mind to peacefully sort out the details of all that has occurred to you, and around you, and allow your mind to develop healthy coping mechanisms for memories from your past; and,

- the universe protects you always, and so it is.

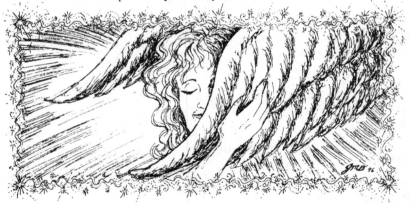

Kendra's words sounded wonderful. I felt as if I were actually pulling myself back together as she spoke. I felt reconnected. I felt safer.

I noticed, as I left the training seminar, it was easier to walk alone outside than it had been. I believed I had been *cured* until I woke-up at 4:00 a.m. again. This time, instead of waking up in the middle of a horrible dream, I woke-up to a sensation of being outside my own body. I was lying in bed, yet I could see myself floating above myself. After a few seconds, I could feel my spiritual self rejoining my physical self. I couldn't help but wonder if it was just my body trying to reintegrate itself.

The next day, I took my first karate class. I thought I would feel safer on the streets if I was better able to defend myself. I hated it. The instructors kept talking about how to inflict injury on assailants and I quickly realized it was not in my nature to do so. I convinced myself to continue going to class—just to learn how to defend myself.

During my second karate class, we were instructed to make the karate yelp noise. Since my assailant had used the same noise when he attacked me, when I heard the noise, it brought back into my mind and body all the feelings I experienced during the attack. In clinical terms, one could say I had attached negative emotions to the sound and that my body reacted negatively when it again heard the sound.

I never went back to class. The incident seriously set-back my recovery. Not only was I continually hearing the sound of the karate yelp, I was also hearing all the negative things my assailant screamed at me during the attack. This went on for about a week until I happened to discuss it with my business associate from *Newbury Hypnotherapy Associates,* Mark Hall.

Mark Hall reminded me of a simple way to *fix* the problem of the sounds in my head.

"Julie, that's easy. If you weren't so tired and stressed-out you would realize that you just have to use a simple NLP technique on yourself."

"Oh?"

"Just put yourself in a trance and turn down the volume of the sounds in your head until you can't hear them anymore. If it turns out you can't do this for yourself, I'll happily to do a session on you, but I'm sure you can do it effectively."

I took Mark's suggestion. It worked immediately. But there was still a problem with going out early or late in the day, and I was still only able to sleep four to five hours at a time.

The following week, I had a breathwork healing session with my friend, William Soo Hoo. As William worked on me, I went into the trance state and felt myself float outside my body. As this occurred, I wondered if William was aware I was outside my body.

After a few moments, I could hear William say to me repeatedly, "It's safe to be in your body; it's safe to be in your body."

As William spoke these words, I came to realize I was waking-up in the middle of the night because I kept leaving my body in the sleep state. I woke-up whenever I re-entered myself.

As William continued to say, "It's safe to be in your body," I allowed my body, mind, and spirit to fully accept this as its truth, knowing as I accepted this truth I would be able to sleep soundly through the night.

When the session was over, William asked me, "Did you know you left your body during the session?"

139

"Yes, I was wondering if you knew."

"I saw it happen."

"I believe I've been waking up in the middle of the night because my emotional self keeps leaving my body in an attempt to feel safe. I wake-up when my emotional self rejoins the rest of me in the middle of the night."

"That's what I was picking-up from the session."

After William worked with me, I was again able to sleep through the night. All I had to do was remind myself, prior to going to bed, that it was safe to be in my body.

The next week, I presented a workshop with NLP master practitioner, James "Jimmy" Green. Jimmy utilized a neurolinguistic programming reframing technique to enable me to ease my remaining symptoms. He placed me in a medium level of trance using simple methods of focus and progressive relaxation. Then, he had me safely and peacefully view the source of my discomfort in a dissociated way. Next, he had me slightly change the scene in my mind until it became tolerable. He instructed me to play the entire scene in my mind, backwards and forwards, repeatedly, changing it and softening it a little bit each time, until it reached a place in my memory where I could be at peace with it.

I left my session with Jimmy Green feeling pleasant but not really convinced that anything had changed. It wasn't until I got home and volunteered to go out for groceries that I realized I was no longer afraid to go outside at night.

Today, only one effect of the attack lingers inside of me. That is, if anyone suddenly rushes up behind me on the street, I mildly panic. I know I could help myself overcome this effect, but I have decided it is in my best interest to allow it to serve me as a self-defense mechanism.

CONCLUSIONS

1. Each practitioner who treated me did so in a loving and therapeutic way. Multiple types of therapy were necessary to restore my mind and body to a peaceful state because the attack affected me on many different levels. While each individual therapy was helpful, none of them would have stood alone (in my case) to bring me into balance.

2. I am now aware, whenever I treat a client for any condition, I should utilize several different types of procedures to foster physical, emotional, spiritual, and psychological wellness.

3. I believe the correct use of a chemical tranquilizer, prescribed by my gynecologist, Dr. Starer, aided me in getting well. I believe the direct and clear advice, suggested to me by Dr. Starer, to seek psychological counseling was sound. For me proper counseling was hypnotherapy, but, had my doctor not made me see the serious nature of the condition I was suffering from, I may not have reached out to others for assistance.

4. When my alcoholic client called me to set-up an appointment (to make-up for his missed appointment), I told him that I had been assaulted and I would no longer be his therapist. I charged him full price for the session he missed and he paid me without balking.

5. As I recovered from the attack, I wrote the book, *Recipes for Wellness*, which is now serving other hypnotherapists across the country. Had I not been afraid to leave my home, it may have taken me years to finish writing *'Recipes'*.

6. The universe provided me with this experience to protect me and to teach me how best to assist others. I now know how to effectively treat victims of violent crime, post-traumatic stress syndrome, and agoraphobia. Had I not been attacked, I would not have the first-hand understanding of these conditions I currently possess.

7. I have never felt more loved, cared for, or protected than I feel today.

Finding Her Way Home
Ending Post Traumatic Stress Syndrome

When I spoke at a health exposition in Northern Connecticut in the Spring of 1995, I didn't know that Monica *(not her real name)* was in the audience desperately looking for words of wisdom to free herself from the torture occurring inside her head. I was there to present group hypnosis seminars, to sell products, and to represent my hypnotherapy training course–not to act as a private therapist. As is often the case, I had no idea how powerfully my words would be received or how much they needed to be heard.

Monica read my program description, *Drawing Love & Prosperity Into Your Life*, and signed up for the class hoping it would make her feel alive again. She had experienced the worst year of her adult life prior to meeting me. Monica had gone to California to help a family member, and in a six-week span of time, fell victim to three traumatic occurrences.

First, she was alone in her sister's home when she heard the sound of breaking glass and realized the property was being burglarized. Fueled by her self-preservation instincts, she quietly moved into a distant area of the house and called the police. The police told her to hide in a closet until they got there and to leave the phone off the hook so they could monitor the home until they arrived. Monica quickly did as the police instructed, but the only sound they heard was her hyperventilating as she hid in the closet.

The police arrived at the scene and apprehended the burglars, but it failed to rid Monica of the terror that plagued her mind. Approximately a week later, Monica was involved in a major earthquake which splintered windows and fractured the building she was in.

Still emotionally fragile from the earthquake and the break-in, three weeks later, Monica became the victim of a drive-by shooting. As she heard the sounds of speeding tires, gunfire, and shattering glass, she cowered to the floorboard of her car and prayed that the bullets would not cause her car's engine to blow-up.

It was of some consolation to her that the police apprehended the gunmen, but the consolation was greatly diminished by Monica's realization of why these men tried to kill her. The police told her the gunmen were out to randomly kill another human being as a gang initiation rite. Her despair in knowing that another human being could view her life (or any life) as being so dispensable seriously crippled her emotions.

Perhaps it was her determination to survive that enabled her to escape from all three of these experiences with only minor surface injuries or, maybe she was being unconsciously granted a second, third, and even fourth chance to be reborn–to start her life over with a new purpose. In any event, she came to me as a victim but quickly became a survivor.

Approximately six months later, I was home in bed on the weekend and almost didn't answer my ringing telephone. After deciding to answer it, I quickly switched into my work mode.

"Good afternoon, The Hypnotherapy Training Company."

"Yes, could I speak with Julie Griffin, please?"

"This is Julie Griffin. To whom am I speaking?"

"This is Monica, Monica Tate. I heard you speak at the expo in April."

"That's lovely, thank you for calling, Monica. What can I do for you?"

"I've been on your mailing list for certification classes and I noticed you changed the location of your classes to Saugus, Massachusetts, from Boston. Are you going to continue to teach in Saugus?"

"Yes, I feel it's a better classroom and easier for people to drive to than Boston."

"I'm very glad you moved. I've had difficulty driving in cities because, last year, when I was in California, I was involved in a drive-by shooting. Things have been really difficult for me since, but I have decided I want my life back. I think taking your course will help me find it. Your seminar, and the tapes I bought from you, have helped me a lot already."

"I'm honored to have been of assistance and I will be more honored to have you as a member of my class. I'm sorry for your trouble."

"Actually, there is much more to it than just the shooting. I can tell you about it in class."

"If you want, we can use you as a subject for learning in class. There is a part of class where I teach hypnosis for overcoming phobias and traumas. If we use you as a subject in class, you will get free personalized therapy while learning how to do the therapy on others."

"I would love that."

"Are you sure? I would not want to invade your privacy."

"I'm sure. I don't need to be private about any of this because I am not embarrassed by any of it. I'd appreciate your help."

"You've got it. It will be wonderful to have such a valid learning experience in class. I'm very sorry for your suffering, but at least now we can change it into a learning experience so it will be of some value."

"I would like that. I'll send in my application form today and I'll see you next week, Julie. I'm glad we got to talk."

"Me too. I'll see you soon. God bless."

ONE WEEK LATER

Monica Tate arrived in my classroom along with my other students. I did not remember meeting her at the expo because I spoke with so many other people that day. Monica was lovely. She readily showed her sweet nature to all those in class. I felt blessed by the opportunity to assist her.

The afternoon of the second day of the class, it came time for us to discuss depression and phobias. I started the class by telling the story of my being mugged and about how all the other therapists assisted me.

As I spoke, there was complete silence in the room. All eyes were on me and it seemed as though the students were so focused on what I was saying that they were forgetting to breathe.

After I completed my anecdotal lesson, I informed the students that I was going to demonstrate therapy to help another person to overcome post-traumatic stress syndrome and its subsequent depression. I started to tell them about Monica's involvement in the drive-by shooting but quickly decided it would be best if Monica told the story.

"Monica, can you tell the story to the class, or is it too difficult to talk about?"

"Actually, I'm glad you asked. I think I need to tell the story."

I had Monica come to the front of the room and take the microphone so everyone would be able to hear her.

As Monica began her tale of woe, I observed the other students tuning-in to what she was saying. Every few minutes, Monica would have to stop to regain her composure. She told the class,

"I felt as if the entire state of California was trying to swallow-me-up, and I kept hearing the sound of glass breaking. There was the sound of glass breaking when they burglarized the house, the sound of glass breaking when the earthquake shattered the windows, and the sound of glass breaking when the windshield of my car was destroyed. The noise keeps replaying in my head."

I passed Monica a tissue and a glass of water so she would be able to continue.

"The thing I find the most difficult to accept about this is that, when the police caught the gunmen, they said they were just out to kill *anyone* as a gang initiation. I can't believe that one human being could perceive the life of another as so dispensable."

Monica broke down again. I asked the entire class to send her love and energy. Monica's state improved rapidly when the class sent her positive energy.

Monica concluded her story. I told the class to take a lunch break and that I would do therapy on Monica afterward. Everyone seemed relieved we were going out for a while. The class was taking the story very personally. I found it impossible not to become emotionally involved.

One of my graduates, Trish Casimira, was retaking the class. She went to lunch with me.

"What are you going to do to help her?" she asked.

"I don't know."

"You don't know?"

"I don't have a clue."

"Should we sit down and figure it out?"

"No, I know it will all come to me when I do the therapy."

"How do you know that?"

"Because it always does. I'm scared right now about this case, because it is really important to me, and, because she is so wonderful. I feel a strong desire to make things right inside her."

"So?"

"If I spend too much time thinking about this outside of therapy, it will make me nervous. I'll say a prayer, ask for guidance, and I will continue to trust that when I start the session, all the right words will come to me."

"That's brave."

"I don't feel brave right now."

THIRTY MINUTES LATER

When class resumed, everyone was anxious to know how I would assist Monica. I suspected the students spent their lunch hour wondering what I would do and feeling grateful they would not have to conduct the session.

As is always the case, as soon as I cleared myself and began the session, I was completely calm, and had no doubts about my ability to assist Monica. I suggested she settle into a comfortable position and I began the session.

"Monica, I'd like you to imagine there is a warm protective blanket being placed around your body and the warmth contained in the blanket is now moving comfortably through your body.

As you enjoy the feeling of warmth moving through your body, I'd like you to focus your eyes on the ceiling as you take in a few long, slow, deep, breaths."

Monica followed my suggestions.

"Monica is it okay if I touch your arms, hands, and forehead during this session?"

"Yes, that's fine."

"You might also feel me at times moving the energy around your body from above you. Is that okay?"

"Yes, that's fine."

"Very good. Continue to feel the warmth of the blanket moving into all the nerves and cells of your body as you focus on the ceiling and breathe in and out. Now, as you exhale, you may allow your eyes to close and allow the closing of your eyes to be a signal for your body to relax completely.

Now, Monica, you may continue to breathe at your own pace, knowing that with each breath you take, and each sound of my voice, you will go comfortably and peacefully into a deeper level of relaxation. Each time you feel me lightly squeeze your wrist, you will go deeper into relaxation. Anytime you feel me gently tap your forehead like this *(I demonstrated the motion)*, you will go into a safe, peaceful place in your mind, and your entire body will function in a relaxed and comfortable way.

Do you understand?"

"Yes."

Monica readily accepted all the suggestions. Her relaxation was apparent as I watched her breathe. The class watched as her body seemed to melt a little with each suggestion I made. There was a visible pulsation showing on one side of her throat.

"Monica, as you relax more and more, you may become aware of the fact that the blanket which is warming you, is also providing you with a barrier of protection. This barrier of protection will help you to remain relaxed and peaceful throughout this session and anytime you think about the incidents discussed during this session. That's right, you now have a barrier of protection surrounding you, and this barrier will continue to protect you emotionally, today and always.

You may also be aware that you are surrounded by the love of everyone in this room. Beyond that, you are surrounded by the love of the entire universe. Everyone in this room will be sending you healing love energy throughout this session. This love energy will be so apparent you may feel as though you are being cradled by angels.

You are feeling your own love and healing energy surfacing. That's right, feel a glow being emitted from your heart. Feel the glow shining brightly, feel it surrounding you. Feel and see in your imagination your own love light forming a protective bubble around your physical being. You may keep this bubble of light around you and know it will always protect your body and soul."

As I held onto Monica's wrist, I could feel small nerve impulses through my fingertips. I sensed she was going deeper into trance when her nerve impulses became stronger and steadier.

I often hold onto the client's wrist throughout a session because the detectable nerve impulses indicate to me how deep the client is, and enables me to connect with the client's subconscious.

As I held her wrist, I telepathically received the following information from Monica's mind and from universal intelligence needed to assist Monica:

◆ Monica's soul is fragmented;

◆ the sound of glass shattering that she continues to hear in her head is representative of the shattering of her soul;

◆ Monica needs to go through a forgiveness process; and

◆ help her!

As quickly as my mind received the information, it went into a mode whereby it instinctively formulates the proper suggestions and analogies. Without hesitation, I continued articulating the therapeutic messages I was receiving from the universe and my own inner-creative mind.

"Monica as you continue to enjoy the relaxed feeling in your body, you may consider the fact that there was a time when forces outside yourself may have seemingly placed you in the position of victim. You may also become aware the victimizers are no longer present in your life. You are safe now and you have decided to move away from thoughts of the past which could potentially continue to victimize you. You have decided to become a survivor because this is your truth. There were incidents in the past which were unpleasant, but you survived them, because you are a survivor.

You have courageously decided to reclaim your life, your happiness, and your freedom. You know you are capable of reclaiming your life, your happiness, and your freedom.

I'd like to point out to you, in doing so, you will be healing yourself. By letting go of anger and despair, you will be creating room inside yourself for love, light, and laughter. By forgiving the past, you can create a dynamic inside your physical being which enables your body to experience its own highest level of health.

You are aware that anger and hate are harmful to your nature, and your health, and that you may choose to forgive the past, and be free of debilitating emotions.

You are also realizing that the real victims in your past have been those who victimized you. Consider what must have occurred in the lives of these victimizers that rendered them capable of such horrid acts. Consider that they, too, are victims–victims of a society that let them down, victims of a less than nurturing upbringing, victims of their own desire to inflict pain upon others. Now they have become victims of themselves, because, as they sowed, so shall they reap."

I stopped giving suggestions for a few moments because I needed to regain my composure. Throughout most of the session, tears rolled down my face. I dried my eyes and took a deep, cleansing breath so I would be clear to speak again.

"Because you believe in doing what is right for yourself and others, you may now choose to forgive all in the past which is helpful and appropriate for you to forgive. You will evaluate which parts of the past were valuable learning lessons. You will learn important lessons from the past that will help you in the future. You will be aware as you learn from the past that you will not have to repeat the unfortunate parts of your life. You know that, because you have forgiven and released the past, you will be free to live in the present–free to enjoy all the beauty in the world.

Among the most important lessons you may learn are:

+ how courageous you are;

+ the universe actually safeguarded you at all times, which is one of the reasons you survived;

+ you are a survivor;

+ you have a very important purpose in the universe and all that occurred in your past has prepared you to fulfill your purpose;

♦   you have a desire to enjoy life which is so strong it enabled you to be here today–it enabled you to reclaim your life, your joy, your happiness; and

♦   you contain all the love and energy inside yourself necessary to fulfill your goals and to manifest your wellness.

Monica, has everything I said registered in your mind and heart as true?"

"Yes."

"Very good. Now, Monica, when I snap my fingers, I would like you to again hear the sound of breaking glass in your mind. It will be different this time. This time you will hear the sound and be able to remain relaxed and comfortable. You will be in total control of the sound as you hear it."

I snapped my fingers. Monica's breathing hastened, so I immediately tapped her forehead so her body would relax.

"You may allow yourself to relax as you hear the sound of glass shattering because you are about to turn the sound down in your head forever. That's right, you are in control of what you allow yourself to hear and what sounds you are capable of turning down or off.

Now, I'd like you to be aware there are sound dimmer switches located on either side of your head, just above your temples. The switches are right here."

I touched the areas I described.

"Now, Monica, as you feel me moving these switches, you may allow your mind to turn down the sound of the glass shattering, and all the sounds that play in your mind as a result of the earthquake, robbery, and shooting. That's right, as I count from one to five, I will be gently moving the switches for you, but it will actually be up to you to turn the sounds down in your head, lower and lower, until you make them disappear. Do you understand?"

"Yes."

"Are you ready to make the sounds go away?"

"Yes."

I began the motion and the count from one to five.

Monica's eyes fluttered as I symbolically made a turning motion at both sides of her head. Her eyes teared as if her mind was experiencing a release of pressure.

"How does that feel?"

"It feels good. It feels like pressure is being released."

"Now, if you are ready, you may say silently along with me the following prayer of forgiveness.

♦ I forgive myself for anything I have done wrong in the past, and I forgive those who have wronged or injured me. I am now free to give and receive unconditional love and to live my life to its fullest. This forgiveness process begins now and continues on inside of me at a healing and appropriate rate.

Very good. And so it is.

Now, Monica, I would like you to scan your mind, your heart, your soul, and your spirit, to see if any of your most important feelings, beliefs, and notions are missing from you. That's right, scan your entire being, and become aware of that which you desire to call back into yourself."

Monica's eye movement indicated to me she was processing my suggestion to scan herself.

"That's right, Monica. Now, I would like you to imagine you are now magnetically drawing back into yourself all the parts of yourself which are helpful and appropriate for you to reclaim. Feel your own personal magnetic force becoming stronger as you fully reclaim what is rightfully yours.

Perhaps you would like to imagine that golden cords of energy are sewing you lovingly back together. Perhaps you would like to feel yourself being surrounded by the love of those in this room . . ."

I then spoke to the rest of the class. "Everyone, please send Monica love, now."

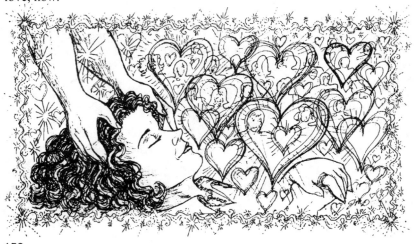

"Feel yourself being embraced by the love freely shared in this room and by the energy the universe is sending down to warm and heal you. Feel yourself becoming complete. Feel your body, mind, and spirit reintegrating, as you again become whole. And so it is.

Now Monica, I would like you to again focus on your heart and allow yourself to feel your own glowing love light. You may allow your love light to continue to grow stronger and brighter each day. This love light will heal, strengthen, protect, and nourish you always.

As you feel your love light growing stronger and steadier, you may say silently to yourself any of the following affirmations which bring you peace or lead you to your highest good.

- I am filled with strength, love, courage, and energy.
- I am now actively healing myself.
- I am now actively forgiving the past.
- All the systems in my body function perfectly.
- I have complete control of my body and my perceptions.
- I am a survivor.
- I am love, light, and laughter.
- I am becoming increasingly comfortable in all surroundings.
- I will only experience fear when it is necessary for my survival. At all other times, I will feel comfortable and safe.
- I am setting goals for myself and moving toward the completion of my goals.
- The light that shines from my heart will grow stronger and brighter each day.
- I eat healthfully, drink water often, and exercise regularly.
- My creativity is steadily surfacing.
- I will put all my talent into practice so I may readily achieve my goals.
- I shall go forth into the world and fully become myself.
- My mind is clear; my heart is full; my soul is free; and I am whole again.
- Each day I will fall more in love with the world around me, as I fall more in love with myself."

As I returned Monica to full conscious awakening, all the students were very still, many were crying. Monica and I held each other for a moment until it became clear to me that Monica wanted to hug all her fellow students. One-by-one, the students embraced her. It was one of the greatest displays of love and sharing I have ever witnessed.

Once everyone settled back into their seats, I allowed time for a question and answer period.

Student #1 asked: Monica, how do you feel?

Monica's response: I feel great. I felt so much love in the room coming from everyone. I know I will be okay now. Thank you all.

The entire class thanked Monica for allowing them to be involved in her process.

Student #2 asked: How did you know what to say to her?

My response: I didn't know what to say at first, but when I touched her wrist and allowed my mind to connect with her's, it became clear to me. I have learned to trust that, when the time comes to help another person, I will automatically receive all the knowledge and insight needed.

Student #3 asked: Where does the knowledge and insight come from?

My response: It is impossible to say for certain, but I believe it comes from many sources, the first being my own inner-creative mind and the second being from the telepathic connection I experience when I work with the client. My third form of assistance comes from universal and spiritual realms.

Student #3 asked: Can you better define universal and spiritual realms?

My response: I cannot define what I do not fully understand myself. In other words, I do not know the exact source of the assistance I receive. It may be spirit guides or angels; it may be from God; it may be information received from a collective universal consciousness. I do not feel a need to know exactly how I know what I know. All I need to do is trust that I will receive all the information I need to assist others and myself. I also consistently take time to give thanks as I receive information.

Student #4 replied: That all sounds very heavy. Do you think this assistance is there for all of us?

I replied: That's a great question. You need to understand a few things. First of all, this information was not shared with me when I took my basic training. I cannot guarantee to you that universal or spiritual assistance occurs, because I cannot prove it. It is up to you to ask inside yourself for assistance (if you want to) and to see if you receive it. I personally believe assistance is available to anyone who asks for it. I do not believe I have been given a gift which is not fully available to anyone who asks for it.

Student #5 asked: This concept of outside assistance does not sit well with me. It sounds frightening and it seems to render you out-of-control.

I replied: I'm really glad you said that, because it gives me the opportunity to remind you that I do not expect you to believe or accept what I am saying as your truth. All I am telling you is that this is my truth. It is up to you to examine your own beliefs and operate in a way which is consistent with *your* beliefs. That is what will make *you* the strongest. If anyone told me when I first started practicing hypnosis I would believe this way, I would have thought he was crazy.

As for your concern about my being out-of-control, let me assure you, I have trained my mind to only speak words which are healthy and healing. My mind and my belief systems are always in control when I speak. The *assistance* is simply available as an all-knowing reference.

Another thing I want to share with you is, as I feel this *assistance* surround me, it is not a scary feeling; quite the contrary. It is, for me, an ultimate feeling of love and protection. It is the same feeling you feel when you know you are with the right mate–it is the same feeling I feel for my love, Roger, and that I share with my brother and sister. It is a feeling of connectedness, of completion.

Student #6 asked: Do you believe your *assistance* is coming from a specific spirit?

I replied: No, I believe it comes from a collective spiritual knowing. I have invited the energy of all that is helpful and good to join me in my work. I believe that is what occurs.

Student #7 asked: So what now, Monica? What are you going to do with yourself?

Monica replied: The first thing I want to do is quit smoking. Can you use me in class tomorrow as a demonstration?

My reply: I'd be honored to. I can also help anyone else here who wants to quit smoking.

Monica continued: When I get home, I'm going to finish my studying, set-up a practice, and hopefully help other people who have been victimized. I think that is what I am supposed to do.

Student #2 asked: Julie, do you think it is appropriate for Monica to try to quit smoking tomorrow with all she is already processing? Wouldn't it be better for her to wait and deal with one thing at a time?

My reply: It is always appropriate for someone to stop smoking. As long as a client wants to stop and asks for help, it is appropriate to facilitate her quitting. It is never appropriate for us to decide a client isn't ready to quit. Monica, are you ready to quit smoking?

Monica's reply: Definitely.

THE NEXT DAY

When class resumed I used Monica as the subject for the stop smoking portion of my teachings. After we finished class, I spent more time working on Monica to reinforce the suggestions given the day before. As I said good-bye to Monica I believed she was okay and I believed she was a non-smoker.

RATIONALE

I used all the techniques on Monica which were used on me (after I was robbed and beaten), that I felt would be appropriate for creating her wellness.

I added the dynamic of having the entire group of students send her healing energy, because it was convenient to do so, and because I have learned the power of group energy.

About three weeks after the class was over I received the following letter from Monica.

Dear Julie,

Enclosed please find my final examination. I would appreciate any feedback you have. I would also like to thank you for your seminar.

You, and the work we did that weekend, gave me my life back. I was tired of trying to make sense of it. I understood logically, but I couldn't feel the logic: I only felt fear, frustration, and horror, a sense of hopelessness.

I had to work, so I chose to work privately for a quadriplegic. After work, I would come home and watch television sitcoms to keep my mind off my reality. I had never even owned a TV until this happened. I always enjoyed reading (anything and everything) but my mind always felt jumpy and I couldn't concentrate enough to read.

Something you said gave me acceptance of what happened. I'm not exactly sure what it was but I am more like my old self—only better. I've been to visit friends, shopped by myself. I go outside and breathe the air and see the beauty and feel joy at being alive. I no longer have to have a few drinks before I go to bed to stop the nightmares and help me sleep and I'm still a non-smoker.

Best of all, I feel I have a purpose in life, which is to help people who suffer as I suffered. I would like to make a difference in the lives of others, as you have made in mine. Again, thank you, Julie, and may love and light be with you always.

Monica

As I read and re-read Monica's letter, I felt the familiar lump forming in my throat that I always feel when I realize something I did made a difference in the life of another human being. I took time to thank the universe for its continued assistance. I allowed my heart to dance in celebration of the joy being a hypnotherapist brings to me.

Not Until the Fat Lady Sings
An Opera Star is Born

" **J**ulie, it's Neil calling." *(Not his real name.)*

Neil is a friend of mine with whom I used to perform. At the time, he was a student at Boston Performing Arts Institute (not a real school). We share a passion for the dramatic and have performed dance and song routines together, publicly, on several occasions.

"Hey, Neil. How's life treating you?

"Great, but I was hoping to partake of your services."

"How so?"

"We are doing an opera at the Institute and I've landed a big part."

"So what is the problem?

"The problem is that I'm not Italian. I can hit all the ranges, but I feel like I'm doing the part a disservice because I can't fully grasp the words I'm singing. When I sing in English, it is easy to put the proper emotion into the words because I understand what I am singing–but this is different. I want to be as inspired in Italian, as I am in English. Can you help me?"

"Sure, I would love to. It will be fun to work on this with you."

"There is one other thing."

"What?"

"I want to do it immediately. Can you fit me in today?"

"If you don't mind coming to my apartment, and if you don't mind that it's a mess."

Since Neil had been in my apartment many times, I felt okay to offer this option. I would have been more formal with a stranger.

"I don't care. You know it doesn't matter to me. I really appreciate your help."

THIRTY MINUTES LATER

Neil knocked on my door.

"Who is it?"

"It's Rocco–Vinny sent me."

FACILITATING WELLNESS

"Get in here, you wise guy.

Neil, is it okay if I use a simple past life regression technique on you? You might not even recall it afterwards. I want to be able to pull up any past life experience you might have had as an Italian."

"That's fine, and while you are at it, could you pull up any past life experience I had as a gigolo? That could come in handy; my expenses are getting tight."

"I wouldn't let you loose on the public. Do you want me to know anything else before we get going, Neil?"

"No, just do it to me, baby."

"I'll do it to you, all right."

"I wish."

"All right, cut the crap. This is a serious thing, and I am a serious person."

"Tell it to someone who might believe you. I must admit though, you looked pretty damn serious singing, 'Love Shack' at Cheers last weekend."

"Neil, look at that nasty crack in the ceiling."

When Neil looked up, I utilized my friend, Roger Meads', method for rapid induction. As Neil looked up, I passed my hand downward in a line with his aura field in the area between his eyebrows. As I did this I said, "SLEEP". Neil immediately went into a somnambulistic trance state. Having worked with Neil previously, I knew a rapid induction technique would work.

I started the session.

"Neil, do I have your permission to touch your arm during this session?"

"You can touch anything, except my penis."

I thought of countless come-backs to his comment, but since he was already under I chose to stop joking around. No matter how well I know a person, once the hypnosis session starts, I don't kid around.

"Neil, each time you feel me squeeze your arm you may allow yourself to go deeper into relaxation. The tenth time I squeeze your arm you will automatically achieve a level of focused relaxation perfect for accepting the suggestions you want to accept."

I moved Neil's arm up and down in a confusing manner, and only squeezed it on every third or fourth movement. By the tenth squeeze Neil's conscious mind had surrendered, and I was fully in touch with the part of his mind I wanted to work with.

"Neil, there are some things I would like to discuss with you, but first, allow me to remind you of your extraordinary performing abilities. I know you know how good an actor, dancer, and singer you are, but it is always nice to be reminded by another person. That's right, Neil–you are a star.

Let's consider for a moment your ability to get into character. I have seen you pretend to be Michael Jackson and obviously you do not really know what it is like to be Michael Jackson or to be inside his body. But you were able to portray Michael Jackson so convincingly it made me want to meet you and perform with you–do you remember? Yet, you are not Michael Jackson–what you are is a performer.

And what is a performer? A performer is someone who portrays another, or who entertains, plays music or sings, or who expresses himself in any live creative way. These are all things you do because you are a performer. You do these things with style, grace, charm, and charisma because you are a performer. These things are naturally inherent in your character because you are a performer.

And how does a performer perform? A performer is able to tap his own inner-creative mind, the inner-creative minds of others, as well as universal consciousness. A performer connects into the all-knowing universal energy field and replicates information inside himself to facilitate his performance. A real performer is capable of becoming the person or thing he is depicting, for a time, by transforming his own energy and creating and/or replicating a new energy. It's all very fascinating, don't you agree?

So the thing is, there is the collective consciousness or universal knowledge–which really is the same thing. This consciousness, this knowledge, is just out there waiting for people like you and me to tap into it. It contains the essence of all knowledge, of all things, and of all times.

You might wonder how you may tap into it. It is simple. All you need to do is to focus on the information or knowledge you want and mentally draw it into yourself. The more you practice this, the better it will work for you.

You may also focus on the abilities of others you would like to replicate inside yourself, and you can draw into yourself the essence of the knowledge and abilities of these individuals. Isn't that wild?

Another important thing for you to be aware of, is that each of us already contains the knowledge of everything there is, inside our own souls. You can find everything you need inside yourself. (By the way, I think all this information is located somewhere between your heart and your mind.)

Neil, I'd like you to relax deeper now as you imagine your mind and spirit are soaring into a higher plane of awareness. That's right, while your body continues to relax, you may allow your mind and spirit to soar into the collective consciousness of the universe so that you may retrieve a profound awareness of Italian.

As I count from one to five your body will become increasingly relaxed and your mind will join forces with the collective consciousness of the universe."

I recited the count.

"Very good, Neil. Now that you are in touch with all knowledge, I would like you to draw into yourself the essence of Italian. That's right, your subconscious will now emotionally understand what it is to be Italian. It will be able to process Italian words and to help you to speak and sing Italian words as an Italian would. Your awareness of Italian will be an unconscious awareness, but it will be perfect for enabling you to perform magnificently in an opera.

Feel yourself drawing in the knowledge of all it is to be Italian, as I count from one to five."

I recited the count.

"Very good. Now I would like you to focus on the talents and abilities of three or four opera stars you would like to have as your own. That's right, focus on these abilities and draw the essence of this talent into yourself, as I count from one to five, knowing you will only be drawing in helpful traits."

I recited the count.

"Excellent. Now I would like you to imagine yourself on stage, performing in an opera. Feel the stage lights on your body and smell the stage make-up on your face. You know anytime you step onto a stage you will go into a state of awareness that enables you to perform your role perfectly.

Notice how casually you are able to be Italian during the performance. Notice how you have blended your own personal style into the styles of your favorite opera stars and how you have created an entirely different, unique style in the process. Don't you look great?

Listen to how marvelously you communicate the language. Notice your pitch and resonance are perfect on every note you sing. Hear the applause coming from the audience. Way to go, Neil.

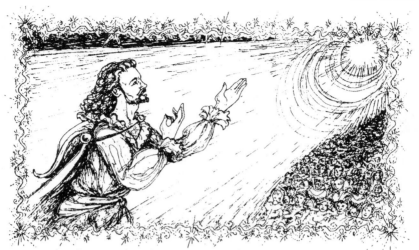

As the curtain closes, you remember how easy it was to be comfortable in your Italian role. You consider how quickly you learned the musical score, and all your lines, and you realize it was because it all felt natural to you.

Now Neil, you may let this scene fade away for a moment, as you get in touch with your own subconscious and inner-creative minds. As I count from five down to one, I would like you to imagine you are walking down a path which leads you to your highest knowing."

I recited the count.

"Neil, you are now in the place inside yourself which has all the answers, all the insight, all the knowledge you will ever require. If it is right and appropriate for you, you may allow your mind to travel backwards in time to another lifetime in which you were Italian. You will only do this if such a lifetime actually existed and only if it will be helpful and safe for you to be consciously aware of such a life.

As I count from one to five, I would like you to imagine you are traveling backward in time, through a warm white light, which will keep you safe and comfortable during your journey. I repeat, you will only have this experience if it is appropriate, safe, and helpful. Otherwise you will continue to stay relaxed and peaceful in the here and now.

One, entering into a warm white light; two, feeling the loving protection of the universe surrounding you; three, feel love and forgiveness emanating from your heart and soul; four, allow your physical and emotional being to remain warm, relaxed, and comfortable; and five, arrive in a past existence, if appropriate.

Now, Neil, you may allow your subconscious to register anything inside this space in your mind which will be helpful for you in your current existence. It is unnecessary for you to have conscious recall of this existence to benefit from it. You will have exactly the kind of knowledge from this experience which is most beneficial to you. You will only recall and retrieve knowledge which is safe, helpful, and appropriate to your fulfilling your highest good in your current life."

I allowed time for his mind to process the experience.

"It is time now for you to travel safely and peacefully back through the warm white light. As I count from five down to one, you will be returning to the current time frame. You will feel warm, safe, peaceful, and relaxed throughout the journey.

Five, moving back through the light; four, feeling warm and relaxed; three, bringing back only helpful knowledge; two, fully reintegrating your body, mind, and spirit in the here and now; and remain deeply relaxed at one.

Neil, I would like you to allow your mind to assimilate all the information you have retrieved from the various processes we have engaged in during this session. Feel yourself assimilating this information, and allow your body and mind to settle down. Allow all the energy in your body to regulate and perfect itself, enabling you to create a perfect state of health in your physical being.

Deeply relaxed, you may say silently to yourself:

- I am a performer.
- I can play any role.
- I can sing any song in any language.
- I have expanded awareness of everything I need to know.
- I actively tap into my subconscious and inner-creative minds.
- I actively tap into universal consciousness.
- I can retrieve data from my subconscious memory banks that will help me in my current existence.
- I radiate charm, charisma, and personal style.
- My voice is clear and resonant.
- I am graceful, striking, and poised.
- I captivate my audience.
- I eat healthfully, exercise regularly, and drink an appropriate amount of water.

- I am not dependent on external things for my health and happiness.
- Joy grows inside me.
- My body is a perfect self-healing mechanism.
- I sleep soundly and awaken rested each day.
- I am a performer.

Very good, Neil. Now you may return to an awareness of the room around you. Come back fully integrated into the here and now at the count of five."

I recited the count.

It took Neil a while to return to full alertness. I allowed him to take his time because there was no rush on my schedule. When he returned, I asked him if he enjoyed the session.

"To tell you the truth, Julie, the last thing I remember is my telling you not to touch my penis."

"That doesn't surprise me."

Tommy: Part One
Pee, Poop & Tommy
Bedwetting Be Gone!

When I met Tommy, he was six years old. His mom brought him to see me, hoping I could help him to get his bodily functions under control.

"The bedwetting thing was bad enough, but now he pees and poops in his pants at school—while he's awake! I can't figure out why he's doing this—why he seems to be getting worse," his mom reported to me.

"I can see how that would be distressing. Is there any abnormal stress going on in your home or at his school?"

"Not that I can think of. He seems to be a pretty happy kid. The only thing I worry about is that he doesn't talk much and he's very shy."

"How shy?"

"Well, he's not as outgoing as his brother and sister. He has friends, but it takes him a while to make friends. When we are out in public, he stays close to me."

"What have you said to him about his peeing and pooping?"

"I asked him why he doesn't wait until he gets in the bathroom and he just shrugs. I try not to get mad about it because I've read it just makes things worse because he gets nervous. But to tell you the truth, it's really starting to wear on me. I used to change the sheets on his bed every night he wet himself, but now I'm finding I only change his bed every two or three days—even if he wets. I've been hoping he will get sick of laying around in his pee and stop."

"Mrs. Grover, I have to tell you, I think that is a big mistake. I know the situation is getting old for you, but the more he sleeps while actively smelling urine the more it will seem natural for him to pee in the bed."

"I didn't think of that."

"I encourage you to clean up after him immediately. Do everything you can to eliminate lingering odors. I will get him under control as quickly as I can so this doesn't remain a problem for long."

"Do you really think you can help him?"

"I'm sure I can. I believe it will be simple, but we will have lasting results if you allow me to see him four times. I'll give you a discounted rate for bringing him in four times. Each session will be a little different. I will tape all the sessions and he will be able to take the tapes home and listen to them in between visits."

I discussed the payment plan and treatment schedule with Mrs. Grover.

"That all sounds very fair and appropriate. I want to go ahead with this. When can you see him—or do you need to see both of us?"

"I think it would be good if you sit in on the first session. Afterwards it will probably be best if I work with Tommy alone—but that is up to you."

"I'd like to come the first time."

We set up a time for the first session.

"Good. Since we are going to do four sessions, I will also be able to help him with self-esteem, confidence, school work, and any other issues that arise."

SESSION ONE

"Hi, Tommy, my name is Julie. Thanks for coming to see me today."

I reached down and shook Tommy's hand. He seemed nervous and shy. He continually looked down and away from me as I spoke to him.

"I'm very happy for you because you are about to learn how to do things which will help you for the rest of your life. I know you are here because you want to be able to control when you pee and poop. Since this is such an easy thing to fix, I will be able to help you with school work and many other things.

I will be giving your mind suggestions which will make you better at all the things that you like to do and will even make school seem easy and fun. I will also be giving you suggestions to only pee and poop when you are at the toilet. Then, you will have control over your body. Is that okay with you?"

Instead of answering me, Tommy looked at his mom for approval.

"You can talk to her Tommy," his mom said.

Tommy blushed.

"I guess it's okay with him," his mom said.

"Good. You will be receiving a tape of today's session and the more you listen to the tape at home, the better the hypnosis will work. I'd like you to listen to this once a day, at whatever time is best for you.

You will be coming to see me a total of four times. I would like you to know that you can get better today. You don't have to wait to take control of your body. You can do it right now. That way, every time you come in, we can celebrate your progress."

I let Tommy know he would get to come in four times, even if he got over his problem the first day. I found early in my practice of working with children, they like hypnosis so much they sometimes delay getting well so they can keep coming to see me.

"Do you understand?"

Tommy nodded to me.

As Tommy and his mom made themselves comfortable, I set up the music and the tape recorder. I began the session by having Tommy imagine he was rocking back and forth on a swing.

"Okay now, I'd like you to imagine you are in a beautiful place and you see a big swing hanging between two tall trees. As you imagine yourself walking closer and closer to the trees, you are relaxing more and more. Now, as you sit on the swing, you relax very deeply. As you enjoy the feeling of the swing swaying you back and forth, and back and forth, you relax completely.

You notice as the swing sways you back and forth, the sunshine is warming your entire body. Enjoy the feeling of the sun's rays relaxing your feet as they move up toward the sky, and feel the sun's rays relaxing your head and face as they move up toward the sky. Feel the sun's rays warming and relaxing the rest of your body as you swing back and forth and as you go deeper and deeper.

I'd like you to imagine as you are swinging, your body is becoming stronger, and your mind is becoming clearer. It's as if you are able to perfectly control your body and focus your mind. As you imagine yourself swinging, your mind is getting smarter, and your body is getting healthier, and you are gaining more control over your body each second. Great.

I'd like you to focus now on any situation in your life which is not working for you, and I would like you to allow your mind to work out solutions to the problem while you are swinging. *(I paused)* Now, I'd like you to picture the situation completely solved. Very good.

I'd like you to focus on anything you enjoy doing and that you want to do better. *(I paused)* Now, see yourself doing what you enjoy doing, well and safely.

Now, I'd like you to see and hear yourself singing, dancing, or playing music. Even if you haven't been doing those things, it is fun to imagine you can. *(I paused)* Don't you sound and look great?

Visualize yourself drawing or painting a picture, or writing a poem, or story. Notice how easy it is for you to be creative and how good you are at creating things. *(I paused)*

Picture yourself doing your homework and getting it done early so you have time to sing, dance, play, and be creative. Doesn't it feel good to get your work done early and to have some free time for yourself? You may notice you even seem to enjoy doing your homework–that suddenly your school work seems fun and interesting. *(I paused)*

You may also notice that the subjects you used to dislike are becoming easy and interesting to you now. Wow! It's almost as if you have the perfect ability to solve problems and to remember things. You notice that when you study and take tests you remain relaxed and you have a wonderful ability to remember things and to answer questions. Isn't that cool?

Now, I'd like you to imagine you can feel energy moving through every part of your body. It feels nice–doesn't it? I'd like you to imagine that the energy is turning a color and the color is making your body work and feel good. That's right–feel the color moving through you, and feel your body becoming perfect. Great job.

Picture yourself getting along with your family, your friends, and your teachers. Notice you are friendly, attractive, nice to be around, and everyone likes you because you treat everyone the way you would like them to treat you. Good.

You know practice is important if you want to become good at something, but you also know that things tend to be easier for you than they are for most people because you are smart and because you have learned how to get your mind and body to work for you.

Each day you will be healthier, stronger, smarter, and more creative. Each day you will have more control of your body.

Tommy, I'd like you to know your mind is now going to tell you when it is time for you to pee and poop. It will tell you in plenty of time so you will be able to make it to the toilet. That's right–your mind is now aware you want to be told when it is time to go to the toilet and your mind will tell you in plenty of time.

When your mind tells you it is time to go to the restroom, you will immediately go. Even if you are sleeping–you will wake-up immediately and go to the toilet. Even if you are at school–you will ask your teacher's permission to go to the restroom–and you will immediately go there.

It will now be easy for you to talk to your teachers, your parents, and all the other helpful people in the world. People like you because you are a nice kid. People want to help you because they care about you.

All the systems in your body are now balancing themselves so you will be able to control when you pee and poop. Your mind is identifying why you used to pee and poop in inappropriate places, and it is now adjusting things inside itself so it will be able to help you to pee and poop at the appropriate times.

Isn't it nice to know you are now taking control over where and when you pee and poop? Won't it be great to wake-up in the morning in dry clothes and in a dry bed? Think how happy you will feel when you can go to school knowing you can control when and where you pee and poop.

I'm very happy for you, Tommy, because the skills you are now learning will help you for the rest of your life. Each day your ability to control your body will increase. Very soon, if not already, you will have total control of when you pee and poop. Excellent!

Now, I'd like you to again feel yourself swinging and relaxing, feeling the sunshine moving through your body as you swing and relax, and feel better each second. Now you may say silently to yourself:

- I am taking control of my body.

- I can control where and when I pee and poop.

- I am proud of my ability to do so.

- Everything is becoming easier for me now.

- I am a great kid. People like me.

- When life becomes stressful, I am able to relax myself and behave appropriately.

- I love life and I love myself.

Excellent. You may imagine your swing is slowing down and you are returning to the here and now. As I count from one to five, you will be returning to this room feeling happy, relaxed, and confident."

When I returned Tommy to full consciousness, he was smiling. I glanced at his mom who had accidentally tranced-out during the session.

"Are you back with us?"

"Yes. I tried to stay alert so I would know what you were saying to him, but I guess I lost it somewhere along the line."

"If you want to know what I said, you may listen to this tape."

I handed her the tape.

"Tommy, you will remember to listen to the tape, right?"

Tommy said nothing. He just blinked.

"Good boy. You did a great job. I'll see you next week. We'll celebrate your progress then, okay?"

Tommy blinked again.

When Tommy went into the other room to get his coat, I quickly told his mother I thought this session would probably cut down the number of his *accidents* 50-75%.

"I think you will see a dramatic reduction in the bedwetting. I am gauging the sessions so he completely stops on the second or third session. This way, his mind will gradually process the changes and the results will be permanent. But, he may surprise me and stop altogether today."

SESSION TWO

Tommy and his mom came in at the appointed time.

"He's doing great. He only had one accident this week."

"Wow, Tommy, that's great, I'm proud of you! Here, let's put a gold star on your folder to show your success. Excellent. Now this week's session will make it even easier to control yourself. What do you think?"

Tommy didn't answer me fast enough to suit his mom.

"I'm sure he's happy about it. You will have to excuse him; he doesn't talk much."

"Tommy, how is school going?"

Again, Tommy's mom answered for him.

"He was in a play this week, right honey?"

"Wow! I bet you were fabulous."

Mrs. Grover then asked me when she should come back to pick Tommy up.

"Give me about 40 minutes."

Tommy's mom left me in charge. When she left, I decided to get Tommy to talk to me.

"So, Tommy, tell me about the play–how did you do?"

Tommy, without hesitation, told me about his part in the play.

"It was a play about a cat and a mouse. I was the mouse. I did good. My teacher told me so."

"I'm sure you did."

"So, what do you think about this hypnosis stuff?"

"It's neat. My friends are jealous of me. They want to get hippotized, too."

I laughed.

"I'm glad you like it, honey. This week's session will be even more fun. Are you ready?"

"Yes."

"Okay, I am going to do things differently this time. I'd like you to sit up on the couch. I'm going to rock you back and forth, if it's okay with you."

He shrugged his shoulders.

"Okay now," I said as I put my hands on his shoulders and had him look into my eyes.

"Now, Tommy, each time I rock you back and forth, you will go deeper into relaxation. On or before the seventh rock, you will be very hypnotized. Look into my eyes, on the third rock you may close your eyes, and you will go under before the seventh rock."

I rocked Tommy back and forth, making sure I had a big smile on my face during the procedure. He followed my directions. On the fifth rock, I felt his muscles let go. I lowered him comfortably onto the couch.

"Very good, Tommy. I'd like you to imagine you are home in your own bed." I said, as I tucked him in.

"Now, as you prepare to go deeper into hypnosis, I would like to tell you a story." I proceeded with the story.

"Once upon a time, there was a handsome six-year-old boy. This boy lives in the town of Stoneham, in the state of Massachusetts, in the country of the United States of America, on the planet Earth. That's right. He is from Earth– not some other planet. He's not from Mars, he's not from Venus. He is an Earthling, a special human Earthling boy, with special human abilities.

And what was so special about this boy, you might ask?

First of all, he had a problem controlling his body, but he got over it completely. That's right, he took complete control of when he peed and pooped and every other function of his body.

It is also easy for him to study and he easily remembers all he studies. He gets along well with his teachers and the other kids at school. Everything about this boy is wonderful.

This boy also gets along well with his family. Even though at one time he was shy, he became increasingly able to talk to people inside and outside his family. Because this boy is nice and kind, everyone likes him. It is easy for him to make friends because he treats everyone with love and respect.

This special boy knows he is as good as anyone else. He knows it will be easy for him to be an athlete, artist, singer, dancer, or anything else he decides to be. He knows he has special abilities which will make his entire life fun and productive.

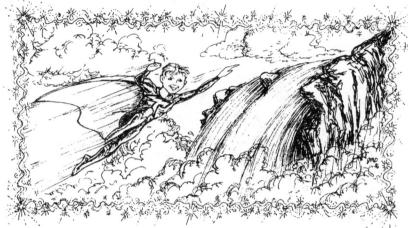

Now, Tommy, I would like you to imagine you are going to meet this special boy who has all the powers and abilities. That's right, I'd like you to meet him.

Where is he? He is in your bedroom; he is in your bathroom; he is in your hallway; he is everywhere you are. Now I'd like you to imagine you are turning around and seeing him. That's right. The special boy is there in the mirror. The special boy with all the power and abilities is you, Tommy. You are the special boy with all the abilities. When you wake-up from this session, you will know you are a special boy with wonderful abilities."

I repeated the most important suggestions from the session in affirmation style and returned Tommy to normal awareness.

"Is that Tommy on my couch, or is it a super-hero?"

Tommy giggled.

His mom tapped on the door. I let her in.

"How did it go?" she asked.

"It was fun, Mom."

"He did fine. Here is his tape. He should listen to this tape a few times, but then let him listen to whichever tape he wants. It really doesn't matter."

TWO DAYS LATER

I received this drawing from Tommy in the mail.

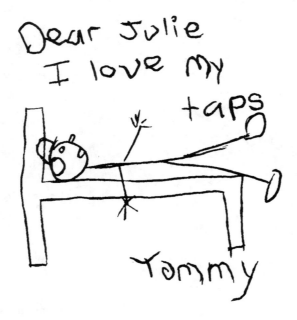

I hung the drawing prominently in my office.

Julie Griffin

Tommy: Part Two
A Visit to Doggie Heaven
Helping a Family Cope with the Loss of A Pet

The next week, when Tommy came in with his mom, I thanked him for the drawing. As he noticed it hanging on the wall in my office, he beamed with pride. Tommy's mom was upset because the family dog, Spotty, had just died. She took me aside and told me she was afraid Tommy would relapse from the stress of losing his pet.

"I wouldn't worry about that. He hasn't had an accident in ten days, right?"

"That's right."

"I think the problem is over. I don't think this will set him back at all. I'll do a session with him today which will help him deal with the dog's passing. What was the dog's name?"

"Spotty."

"How did Spotty die?"

"He had been sick for about a month. He was very old. My husband and I had him put to sleep last night."

"I'm very sorry."

"It's tough to take. We had Spotty for twelve years–that's six years longer than we've had Tommy."

I realized that Tommy's mom was having more trouble with the dog's passing than Tommy was.

"Mrs. Grover, why don't you sit in on the session with us today. It's going to be about Spotty. I think you will like it."

"Okay, that sounds good."

I passed her a Kleenex and asked them both to settle in.

I asked them to take long, slow, deep breaths along with me until I was certain they were relaxed and focused.

"Okay now, I'd like you to imagine it is summer again and you are at home sitting in front of the lake. You feel very relaxed and peaceful as you go over and lie down in the most comfortable lounge chair. You continue to relax more and more as you watch the clouds passing by in the sky. You continue to

173

go deeper as the sunshine kisses your skin with its warmth. You may notice the sun is helping your body to melt into relaxation. As you relax more and more, you hear a wonderful message playing in your head and the message says, 'sleep . . . sleep . . . sleep . . . ' As you allow yourself to drift off to sleep you have a wonderful dream. In this dream, you have been given a key. When you ask what the key is for, you are told the key unlocks the gate to Doggie Heaven.

You are very happy because you know Spotty is in Doggie Heaven and you are looking forward to seeing him one more time. As you walk down the path to Doggie Heaven, you notice dog biscuits are growing on all the trees and the road is lined with Frisbees. When you get to the gate, you are very surprised to realize that all the dogs in Doggie Heaven have extraordinary abilities. All the dogs in Doggie Heaven can talk and drive cars.

There is a dog named Great Dane at the gate, dressed in a tuxedo and wearing a top-hat. He asks you to use your key. You take your key and unlock the gate and it swings open for you to enter.

'Oh, my goodness, you are live human beings! What in heaven's name are you doing here?' Great Dane asked.

'We are here to see Spotty Grover. Is he here?'

'Spotty Grover? Of course he's here. He's a great dog! Where else would he be? Just a minute, I will call him for you. I think he's down at the lake playing with Polly Poodle.'

Great Dane got on the intercom and announced,

'Attention, Spotty Grover. You have visitors from Earth. I think they are your family. They look like nice people, but I don't think they have any toys with them. Please proceed to the golden gate to greet your visitors.'

You notice how beautiful everything is in Doggie Heaven. It's warm, the air smells wonderful, there is a lake with flowers growing around it and bunny rabbits and squirrels are hopping about.

A bunny rabbit hops up to you and says, 'Hi, Tommy. My name is Furry Rabbit. Spotty sent me down to tell you he will be here to see you in just a minute.'

You are surprised the bunny is not afraid of Spotty, but Furry Rabbit tells you, 'It's okay, Spotty is my friend. All the animals in Doggie Heaven are friends.'

Suddenly, you see Spotty arriving in his own private boat. You notice how different he looks, but you are sure it is Spotty. He runs up to you and drops a ball on your lap and lays a wet sloppy kiss on your face. His tail is wagging, and he has a wonderful glint in his eyes. You notice Spotty looks young and healthy. You ask him why he looks so young.

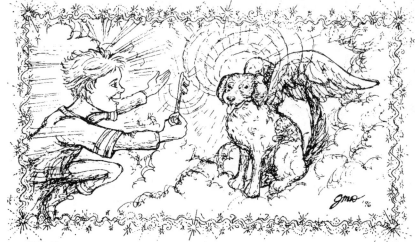

'Well, Tommy, it's because, when you go to heaven, you get to be all better again. No matter what you have gone through in life, you get to be perfect when you go to heaven. I'm glad you came to see me, Tommy, because I want you to know that I am fine and, even though I will miss you, it is better for me to be here because I feel good again. You will always be in my heart. I love you, Tommy; please tell everyone I am fine.'

I ended the session by restating that Tommy would continue to be in control of his body and to gain confidence.

When I concluded the session, Tommy's mom gave me a hug.

"I don't know about Tommy, but the session made me feel better."

"I'm glad."

THE NEXT DAY

Tommy's mom called and told me the entire family had listened to the tape of the session together.

"It helped all of us. Even my husband liked it. Thank you."

I did one last session with Tommy. We again celebrated his success with gold stars on his folder and by playing a song on the electronic keyboard in my office. Each time he came to see me, he was less shy, so I decided to report this to his mom.

"Tommy is very chatty with me now. It is only when you are here that he clams-up. I know you are trying to make things easy for him, but I think it is important you give him time to speak for himself. He can do it. Thanks for bringing him in to see me. You have done a wonderful job with him. It has been great having him here. I love him."

"It shows."

Vomit and Tommy's Sister Tammy
Getting the Butterflies Out of Tammy's Tummy

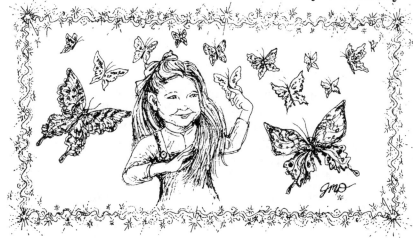

A couple of months after Tommy's therapy was over, his mom called me. "Hi, Julie. It's Ann Grover."

"Hi, Mrs. Grover, how are you?"

"I'm fine, and for goodness sake, call me Ann. After all we have been through, I feel like you're a part of my family."

"Thank you. How is Tommy doing?"

"Just great. He's only had one accident in the last two months."

"How did you handle that?"

"I just said, 'OOPS!' to him in a relaxed manner and we never discussed it beyond that. I think it was just a fluke. He still listens to your tapes every few days. I don't make him do it, he just does it. I'm sure he's fine."

"That's nice to hear. I appreciate your calling to let me know."

"Actually, Julie, that's not what I'm calling about."

"Oh?"

"I'm calling about my daughter, Tammy."

"Tammy? She's your eleven-year-old?"

"Yes, you have a good memory."

"What may I do to help Tammy?"

"She became ill just before her last three exams."

"Would you describe the nature of the illness to me, please?"

"She threw-up each time."

"Is this new behavior for her?"

"Yes. She has always worried unduly about tests, but throwing-up is new."

"Is she struggling at school?"

"On the contrary. She is an excellent student–straight A's. I fear she is overly concerned with being perfect. I hope I haven't made her think she has to be perfect."

"You are an excellent mother, but you might want to relax more. Practice letting go of your stress and concerns so they don't inadvertently trickle down to the kids. It will only improve your already excellent parenting skills."

I spoke these words to Ann after registering she was aware of the fact that this was the second child she was bringing to see me who had trouble controlling bodily functions. I knew she had already realized that since two of her three children had similar problems, she might inadvertently be creating a dynamic inside the kids which caused these reactions.

"Do you think you can help Tammy?"

"Not only do I know I can help Tammy, I think it will be easier than it was to help Tommy. I can't be sure until I meet with her, but I think it should only take two sessions."

"Really? It seems so violent when it occurs."

"All I have to do is to give her suggestions that her belly and all other parts of her body will be calm when she studies, when she takes tests, and at all other times. There are a few other dynamics I will incorporate as well."

We set-up a time for me to meet with Tammy. Ann decided to let Tammy have both the sessions alone with me. I was happy about her decision, as it afforded me the opportunity to privately question Tammy.

THE APPOINTMENT DAY

When Tammy came into the office, she was clearly excited to meet me. She was a pretty, slender girl, with a meticulous appearance.

"Tammy, your mother showed me pictures of you, but you are much more beautiful in person."

"Thank you," she said as she blushed.

"Did your mom tell you she wants me to hypnotize you?"

"Yes."

"How do you feel about that?"

"I think it's awesome. I listened to the tape about Spotty and I really liked it. I'm glad my mom brought me here."

"Good. Now your mom tells me you have been having trouble with your belly before you take tests. Do you know why?"

"No, I didn't even realize I threw-up every night before tests until my mom pointed it out to me. I don't mean to do it."

"I'm sure you don't. I just want to help you relax so you will be comfortable in the future. Okay?"

"Sure."

"I want to ask you a few questions first. How is school going?"

"It's fine. I like it."

"How is everything at home?"

"It's good, too."

"Has anything been bugging you?"

"Not that I can think of; I just want to make sure I keep getting A's because I heard my parents talking about how good it would be if my sister and I get scholarships. I don't want to let them down."

"I'm sure you will never let them down. I don't think they expect you to get all A's, do you?"

"I don't know."

"Besides, it is really easy for you to get A's, isn't it?"

"Yes, I guess so."

"Your mom told me that not only do you get all A's but you usually get 100%. That is very impressive. Do you realize you would still get an A even if you got one or two things wrong?"

"Really?"

"Yes, you only need to get 93% to get an A. I think you will still get everything right because you are naturally smart and because you study, but it would be fine if, under some strange circumstance, you did something less than perfectly. Nobody expects you to be perfect. Your parents will always love you and be proud of you no matter what.

Tammy, is there anything else you want me to know or to help you with while you are here? I'm happy to talk with you and to help you."

"What do you mean?"

"You are here today, plus you will be coming in one more time. I'm sure we can straighten out your belly today, so if there is anything else you want help with, we can do that, too."

"Can you help me to play the flute perfectly?"

"I would be happy to help you to play the flute better, but, please remember, you do not have to do things perfectly. It is okay to do things in a way that is comfortable and fun; it is okay for you to enjoy being a kid."

"Okay."

"Is there anything else you want me to know?"

"No. That's all."

"Tammy, is it okay with you if I touch your arm and hand during the session?"

"Sure."

I explained to Tammy how hypnosis works and I asked her to breathe and relax along with me. I had her imagine her body was melting into relaxation as she swung back and forth on a hammock. Next, I had her imagine she was on top of a beautiful mountain and she was going deeper into relaxation as she walked down the mountain. Once she was deeply relaxed, I gave her the following suggestions:

- Focus on the areas of your body that most need to relax, and feel those areas melt into relaxation.

- Feel relaxation moving and flowing through your entire body, but especially through the areas where tension tends to accumulate.

- Feel relaxation flowing through those areas and command your body to keep these areas relaxed always–no matter what is occurring, no matter what is going on, no matter what you are doing, relaxation will always flow through these areas so you will be able to focus on whatever you are doing in a peaceful, clear, and alert manner.

- Know anytime you sit down to study or to take a test that relaxation will automatically flow through your body, and your mind and it will help you to remember things.

You are now aware that each time you sit down to study or to take an exam that your mental powers will become more profound, more concentrated, and more effective.

Become aware that anytime you place your index finger and thumb in a circular position on either or both of your hands, this will be your mind's cue to relax, and to store and recall information. This process will work for you everywhere you go."

I reached over and moved her thumb and index finger into the circular position I described.

"Anytime you place your thumb and index finger in a circular position your body will relax, your mind will become clear, and you will be able to store or access information inside yourself.

The more you practice doing this, the better it will work for you. Soon it will become an automatic process. Soon you will automatically place your fingers in this position anytime it is appropriate for you to go into a relaxation or learning mode. It will simply happen and you may enjoy the process as it occurs.

From now on, you will feel more and more comfortable with your ability to learn, to solve problems, to see patterns, and to ascertain solutions. Learning, studying, and even exam-taking will become challenges you enjoy. You will find the closer it comes to the time of an exam, the more relaxed and confident you will be of your ability to pass your exam with a high level of competency.

Your ability to play the flute is now improving, too. Your hands connect wonderfully to the flute. Your fingers move with precision on the keys of the flute. When you play the flute, it is as though you can feel music flowing down from heaven, into your soul, and coming out through your flute. You play music beautifully because you are a musician. You enjoy playing the flute and you feel relaxed and happy when you play.

You derive great pleasure as you see yourself becoming more confident and effective each day. It almost seems as though you have released feelings of love and happiness inside yourself. You know you are greatly loved by all those around you. You know your future is secure and you will be able to attend college, if you so desire.

Your mind is now putting all your thoughts in order. Your mind is now working so that you may feel peaceful and confident. Your mind solves problems inside itself and helps you to develop healthy coping mechanisms for everything which occurs around you.

Your body functions wonderfully for you. You eat healthfully, exercise regularly, and drink water appropriately. You stop and notice how beautiful the world is. You feel relaxed and happy each time you see the blueness of the sky. Each day you will feel happier, healthier, and more creative.

As Tammy returned to full consciousness, I wrote her a note and stuck it in the case of her audio cassette. The note read:

Dear Tammy,

Keep up the good work and have fun in the process.

Love,

Julie

I gave Tammy the tape, told her to listen to it a few more times and that I would see her the next week. I asked her to bring her flute to the next session.

ONE WEEK LATER

Tammy arrived at my office and proudly reported that she remained comfortable the entire week, even though she contended with two major exams.

After congratulating her, I did a simple reinforcement session. After the session, I asked her to play me a tune on her flute.

"I only know one song by heart, but I can play it for you. It's called Joy."

Tammy's song moved through my heart and touched my soul.

Her Soul's Emancipation
Freedom From A Dysfunctional Marriage

I worked with Veronica Vanderkelen *(not her real name)* in my creative arts and athletic programs. I knew her to be an excellent hypnotic subject and an upbeat person. I was sad to hear she needed a completely different type of therapy.

"Julie, it's Veronica Vanderkelen," she said, sounding desperate.

"Hello, Veronica. What's wrong?"

"I'm a mess; I need help. I've left my husband, but I'm afraid I will go back to him if you don't hypnotize me into staying away from him."

"Are you sure that you want to leave him? You two always looked like the perfect couple."

"Looks are very deceiving in our case. I have been trying to leave him for the last two months. He keeps using emotional blackmail to get me to go home, but not this time. This time too many lines have been crossed. I can't go back."

"May I ask you what lines have been crossed?"

"I found out he's been sleeping with my so-called friend, Terri, in our own bed, when I go away on business."

"Ouch. I'm sorry, Veronica."

"What hurts the most is all the lying. He has been telling me for months that he wants to save our marriage—begging me to stay with him—all the while he's screwing someone else. I don't get it."

"I would not have guessed any of this."

"I know. No one knew the truth about how on edge we have been for the last year. But I can't take it any more. I want to be happy; I want to be with someone I can trust. Can you help me stay away from him?"

"Veronica, I can help you to relax, and to think clearly and act in your own best interest, but I cannot suggest that you will not go back to him. I can help you to let go of the past and to move in the direction of your highest good, but I cannot suggest to you what your highest good is because I do not know what it is."

"That makes sense, Julie. I respect that. I will be able to stay away from him if you give me suggestions like those because I am sure it is right to leave him. I have been praying for a sign to tell me whether I should leave or stay. I don't think I could have gotten a clearer signal than this."

"Okay, you sound clear and reasonable in your choice. When do you want to come in?"

"May I come in first thing tomorrow morning?"

"I can see you at 9:00 a.m."

"I'll see you then."

THE NEXT MORNING

Veronica came in looking as if she hadn't slept in days.

"Hi, come on in." As I gave her a hug, Veronica broke down into uncontrollable sobbing.

"I'm sorry, Julie. I get into these crying fits and I can't seem to stop."

"You shouldn't try to stop. Crying is a healthy healing mechanism."

"But I'm afraid the pain will never go away."

"Another hypnotherapist, Katie Ellis, once told me, the deeper the pain, the deeper the healing. I think it's true. You are much better off acknowledging the pain and grieving it honestly. Then you will be free to move into the future without it."

"What do you mean?"

"I treat a lot of clients for drug and alcohol addiction and even for weight loss who are eating, drinking, or using drugs to try to cover-up a feeling of pain inside themselves. They don't realize eating, drinking, and using drugs will never take the pain away."

"So what will?"

"Crying will. I believe you should acknowledge your pain, see what lesson you learn as a result of it, grieve appropriately by crying, release the despair, and allow love to fill the void. I think, until you actively go through this grieving and releasing process, you will carry the pain and sadness around with you, as if it's your own private anchor."

"So what can you do for me here today?"

"I can do a relaxation session which will help you to sort out your feelings and to take positive steps toward your best future. It will be up to you to identify what that future will be and what steps you need to take, but I'm sure this session will facilitate the process."

"Okay, the sooner the better," Veronica said as she climbed into my recliner. "I hate feeling like this."

I grabbed a comforter and placed it over her. I generally ask permission to do this, but Veronica clearly needed to be babied so I just did it. Even though Veronica always presented herself as strong and confident, I could see she had been deeply wounded by the betrayal of her trust by her husband and friend.

"Veronica, may I touch your wrist and forehead during the session?"

"Touch away."

I had Veronica begin her session by breathing long, slow, deep breaths along with me. *I often begin a session this way because it enables me to get on the same wavelength as the client.* I gave her a suggestion that, anytime she felt me squeeze her wrist, she would go deeper into a feeling of peaceful comfort.

Veronica went into a deep trance almost instantly. I was mindful not to allow her to go too deep because I wanted her to process the session in a fairly alert state of trance.

As Veronica reached the desired depth level I was reminded of therapy techniques hypnotherapist Peter M. Rogine utilized on similar cases. I reached deep inside my memory banks and turned on my own inner-creative mind so I could retrieve his teachings and process them in a way which would serve Veronica. Much of the therapy utilized in this case is my interpretation of Peter Rogine's techniques.

"You may now go into a safe place inside yourself. That's right. Find a path inside yourself which leads you to your own truth. Find a safe, secret place which is only yours. As you find yourself on this path, I'd like you to become aware of a wonderful healing energy you are now generating inside your fingers and hands.

Feel a wonderful, warm, and gentle electric current moving through your hands and fingers. Feel it traveling up your arms and moving very slowly and comfortably through the rest of your body. Now you may take your hands and place them on your heart and allow the healing energy inside your hands and fingers to travel into the deepest corners of your heart. Allow that energy to move through your heart and into your soul as you drift deeper and as you find yourself in a safe and secret place inside yourself. Very good.

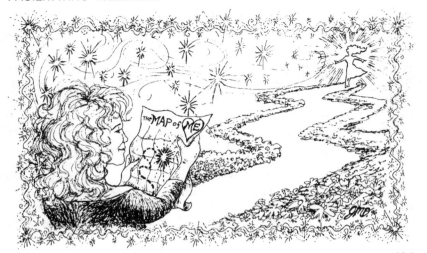

Feel your entire body relax as you picture yourself outside in a beautiful place. Picture yourself in a garden and notice there are two small tables in this garden. You are relaxing more and more as you allow yourself to go over to the first table. On this table you notice there is a small blank book. I'd like you to notice that on the cover of the book you may read the words, *THE BOOK OF SADNESS*.

Now, I would like you to pick up *THE BOOK OF SADNESS* and imagine you are writing inside it all the disappointments of your entire life. That's right, see yourself writing in all the old hurts, the despair, the issues which can never be resolved, the grief, and any other emotions, thoughts, or details of the past which might prevent you from moving freely into a happy future.

That's right—jot down the dreams you had which you know will never manifest. Write it all down and notice how with each entry you make into *THE BOOK OF SADNESS,* you feel freer. That's right; you feel a sense of relief with each notation you make. Good.

Next, I would like you to notice there is a large deep hole in the ground and a shovel next to it. I would like you to picture yourself walking over to the hole in the ground and dropping *THE BOOK OF SADNESS* into the hole.

Next, you may pick-up the shovel and begin the process of burying the sadness of the past, one shovel full at a time. That's right; at your own pace you will be able to let go of the past and to bury it one shovel full at a time.

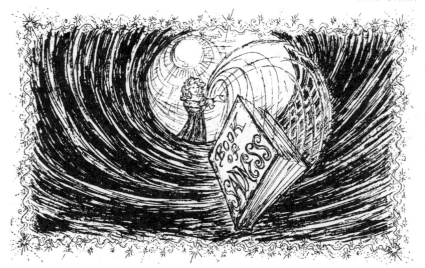

I would like you to know, one day soon you will look up into the sky and see a sign that tells you it is time to finish burying the book.

Now, imagine the book has already been buried and take some time to examine the positive lessons you learned from your past. I would also like you to consider that no matter what occurred in the past, you managed to survive it because you are a survivor. Realize too, all the steps you took in the past have made you who you are today, and the person you have become is truly a wonderful gift to the world.

You may become aware that you have learned positive lessons from your past and you will now be able to move freely and joyously into the future. Wonderful.

Now, I'd like you to notice on the second table there are two bags. The first bag is full of grass seed. I would like you to see yourself sprinkling the grass seed over the fresh pure earth that covers *THE BOOK OF SADNESS.* Feel yourself pressing the seeds into the ground with your feet.

Notice that the second bag contains three tulip bulbs. I'd like you to plant the red tulip bulb, knowing it represents the positive love which is about to grow in your heart and which you will find inside of life itself.

Now, you may plant the yellow tulip bulb, knowing it is representational of the positive health you will continually manifest in your body.

And, you may plant the violet tulip bulb, knowing it represents the positive life you are about to build for yourself.

You are fully aware you have planted positive love, positive health, and positive life in the garden of your mind and these very things have already begun to grow inside you. Very good.

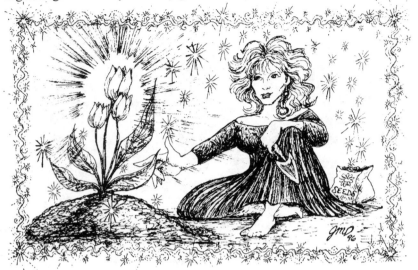

Veronica, I'd like you to relax deeper as you become aware each time you face your past, learn from your past, and let go of your past, you are creating room inside yourself for love and happiness. You may go deeper into relaxation as you consider this, and as you feel love and joy growing inside you.

You may notice there is a second book on the first table in the garden. I'd like you to imagine you are picking up this second book and noticing the cover reads, *THE BOOK OF YOUR FUTURE,* but all its pages are blank.

There is a very important reason the pages are blank and it is because it is up to you to decide your own future. You may now decide to repeat the past, or to learn from it and take what you have learned into a brighter future. It's your choice, and you can begin the process of making all the right choices now, choices which will ensure your happiness, your health, and your total fulfillment.

I'd like you to picture yourself writing the chapters of your future. Write about how you want your life to be and how you will make it so. Picture yourself writing down your highest truths and all the things you will tell yourself to enable you to achieve your highest good. That's right. Write yourself as the heroine of the story and be sure to write a happy ending because you are now creating your future in your mind.

Now, I'd like you to picture yourself walking up a hill and feeling lighter and freer with each step you take. Feel the sunlight kissing your skin with its warmth; feel the gentle breeze putting wind inside the sails of your soul. Feel the flow of the universe carrying you into a better place–a place where you will be free to become all you desire and deserve to be.

Imagine you are becoming a part of the sky, a part of the path you walk upon. Know you are the best parts of all that is beautiful. You are like the scent of a rose, like its hue. You are like it as it blossoms and blooms; you are all its celebrated parts.

As you realize this, you may begin your process of self-celebration–a joyous celebration of all you are and all you are about to become.

Celebrate your own vital place inside the flow of the universe knowing that, as you feel part of the universe, you will never feel alone.

Now, Veronica, feeling relaxed and clear, you may allow these sentiments to echo inside you:

- I am learning from my past and releasing all thoughts and energies which are not in line with my highest good.

- I am releasing myself from religious programming that is inappropriate to my highest good.

- I am forgiving myself for anything I have done wrong, and I am forgiving all those who have injured me.

- I am now free to give and receive unconditional love and to experience joy to its fullest.

- I consistently think clearly and act in my own best interest.

- I shall rise up and move forward.

- I operate inside the flow of the universe.

- I am the flow of the universe.

- I am allowing the universal flow to move me toward my highest good.

- One day soon, I will look up into the sky and see a sign that clearly lets me know which way to go.

- I have all the strength, courage, and creativity needed to get me through this day, and all the days of my life.

- I will continue to eat healthfully, drink water, exercise, to meditate or pray, and to count my many blessings.

- My mind is clear; my heart is full; my body heals; my soul is free; and I will be happy."

I slowly returned Veronica to full conscious awakening. I allowed her to remain relaxed while I rewound the tape of the session.

"Veronica, I taped this session. I think it will be helpful for you to listen to it several more times. It will help you to grieve for all the disappointment you have had recently as well as for past disappointments. It will also help you to sort out what to do with yourself now."

"Julie, I feel much more relaxed, but I still feel like crying."

"I would be worried about you if you didn't feel like crying. Think of tears as your friends right now. Keep listening to this tape and keep crying until you are all cried out. Then you will really be able to start living again. I promise. I think it would be a good thing if you come to see me again in about a week. Do you want to?"

"Yes, I think I do."

ONE WEEK LATER

Veronica came to see me. She was still crying a lot.

"Have you been listening to the tape?"

"Yes, Julie. I listen to it every day. I know it is helping me to think clearly. But there is one thing going on that is really disturbing me."

"What is that?"

"I keep dreaming about them."

"Dreaming about who?"

"About Steve and Terri."

"Do you want to tell me about the dreams?"

"I think I need to tell you. I keep dreaming he is making love to her in my bed. I see him giving her all the affection I begged him for. I see them plotting the lies they told me."

"How do you feel about the dreams?"

"I wake-up screaming from them. Now I even feel like I have the dreams when I'm wide awake. It's strange, I can be walking down the street and suddenly a flash of them having sex runs through my mind and I start screaming. Have you ever heard of such a thing?"

"It sounds like a flashback, only you are flashing back to something you never actually saw. You never actually saw them together, did you?"

"No, but you are right; it is like I'm flashing right into something. Why do you think this is happening?"

"Veronica, I'm not a psychologist. I can't guess or suggest what may be going on. What I can do is relax you, and when you are hypnotized, I can ask you why this is occurring."

"How will that work? If I am not able to tell you why it's happening now, why do you think I will be able to tell you when I am hypnotized?"

"This may be difficult to understand, but a part of your subconscious creates your dreams and is now creating the daytime flashes because it is trying to help you to sort through your life and to make the right decisions. I don't know why your mind is showing you these pictures, but I'm sure deep inside yourself you know why."

"Wow. That's heavy."

"I guess what you have to decide is if you are ready to consciously know what your mind is trying to tell you."

"I have to know. I can't live like this. I have to make decisions about my life. I can't keep living in the back room of my office and pretending everything is okay when I really feel like a big piece of me is dying."

Veronica started to sob again.

"You mean you haven't told anyone you left Steve?"

"Almost no one."

"Why not?"

"I'm ashamed, embarrassed, hurt, humiliated. I can't discuss this without going to pieces. I don't want anyone else to see me this way. For Christ's sake, I'm a counselor. Things like this aren't supposed to happen to me."

"Veronica, there is no shame in what you are going through. In fact, what you are doing takes a vast amount of courage. You could have just run back to him and pretended it didn't happen. But, instead, you've found the courage it takes to step aside and clearly examine what is best for you for the long haul. I'm very proud of you. No matter what you decide to do, I'm proud of you."

"Thanks. I've never looked at it that way. I guess it's the old Catholic guilt. Part of me thinks it is wrong to leave my husband, no matter what he did."

"Veronica, did you hear what you just said?"

"Yes, I heard it, and I know how ridiculous the statement is. It's just that my mother's life sucked–but she never left my dad. My grandmother's life sucked–but she never left my grandfather. I feel like I'm betraying all of that."

"You might want to ask yourself who you will be betraying if you go back to a life which is not appropriate to your highest good. You need to ask yourself if it would serve you or Steve if you return to him."

"You're right. I would be betraying myself for absolutely no reason because the marriage was not working for either one of us. No matter how much glue you use, a shattered teapot is never going to hold water."

"Good analogy, my dear."

"That's actually not the best analogy I have come up with lately."

"Oh?"

"Since I found out about the affair I have developed my first case of hemorrhoids. Apparently, this situation has given me a flaming pain in the ass."

"Veronica, as long as you keep your sense of humor you are going to be okay. Let me tuck you in so you may take a nice long trip to Trance-L-Vania. This session will be different than what we usually do because I'm going to ask you questions when you are under. Is that okay with you?"

"'A girl's gotta do what a girl's gotta do.'"

I induced trance by asking Veronica to breathe deeply while I made passes in a downward direction in line with her aura. I had her imagine warm waves of beautifully colored energy moving across her body as I made the passes. I could see her relaxation increase with each pass I made.

After about a dozen passes, I suggested she find herself moving back into the secret place inside herself that has all the answers. I told her she could contact her own higher self. I suggested she would be able to safely and peacefully identify reasons for all she was doing and creating.

I told her, as I counted from one to ten, she could imagine herself walking farther into her own highest knowing and, at the number ten, she would be able to answer any of the questions I asked her, provided it was in her best interest to know the answers to the questions. I also told her with each higher number she would feel increasingly relaxed and euphoric.

I recited the count and watched her physical reactions, to be certain she was responding in a favorable way to the suggestions. At the number ten, I began to directly question her.

"Veronica, when you came here today, you told me you have been having very disturbing dreams and conscious flashes which are similar to the dreams. If your subconscious is aware of these dreams and flashes, I would like you to indicate so to me by raising your *yes* finger." *(I had previously programmed yes and no ideomotor response fingers with Veronica. I was aware that when she rapidly raised her right index finger that was her subconscious mind's ideomotor yes response.)* Veronica's *yes* finger immediately raised.

My first mentor, Marie Cowden, introduced me to the helpful use of ideomotor finger response. I often work with ideomotor finger signals in addition to verbal response techniques, so I then said:

"Veronica, if your subconscious is aware of the reason you have been having the nightmares and flashes, you may now say 'yes' to me verbally."

Veronica immediately responded, "Yes."

Since both the verbal and ideomotor responses matched, I was convinced her subconscious had the desired information, so I continued to ask more questions.

"Veronica, can you tell me why your subconscious has been presenting you with these dreams and flashes?"

"Yes. My mind does not want me to forget the betrayal. My mind knows I must leave Steve, so it is going to keep reminding me of the betrayal until it is certain I will leave him forever."

"Why does your mind want you to leave Steve?"

"Because there is no longer a purpose left for us to be together. We cannot help each other any further. All we do is hurt one another. My mind does not want me to stay out of loyalty, so it is showing me repeatedly he does not deserve loyalty."

"That makes sense to me, Veronica. Does it make sense to you?"

"Yes, it makes perfect sense."

"Veronica, now that you know the purpose of your mind showing you these pictures, are you going to be able to do the right thing for yourself or should your mind keep reminding you of this?"

"What do you mean?"

"Should we tell your subconscious that you fully understand this message and it may allow your mind to rest now?"

"Yes. I don't want to keep seeing those pictures."

"Okay. Your mind is now becoming aware that you have received the message and you will now act wholly and fully in your best interest.

Veronica, I am going to start a sentence, and, when I tap your forehead, I want you to complete the sentence. Are you ready?"

"Yes," Veronica said, as her 'yes' finger jumped.

"If I had it all to do over again, I would . . ."

I tapped her forehead.

" . . . I would do it all over again," Veronica said, as tears rolled down her cheeks.

I was very surprised by her response. It made me wonder if she unconsciously wanted to go back to her husband. I knew I had to find out.

"Veronica, you just stated, 'If I had it all to do over again, I would do it all over again.' Would you please elaborate on this response and tell me what it means in the grand scheme of things."

I was very careful as to what I said because I did not want to inadvertently suggest to her what she was thinking.

I tapped her on the forehead to gain her response.

"It means I am not sorry I married Steve. We had twelve years together and ten of them were good years. Some people never have the opportunity to enjoy ten years with someone they love. I'm glad you asked me the question about doing it all over again. It made me realize, despite everything, a part of me still loves him and is grateful for all we shared."

"So what do you want your future to bring to you?"

"A new life, without him. I know I must leave him. Our time together is over. I'm supposed to be somewhere else now."

I breathed a sigh of relief. I know as a hypnotherapist I must keep my opinions to myself at times like this, but a part of me wanted to stand up and applaud her choice. I did not want her to go back to Steve. I knew them both, and I knew she deserved more than he was giving to her.

Veronica, I'd like you to relax more deeply. I'd like you to imagine you are melting into perfect, peaceful, relaxation. Perhaps you'd like to imagine you are a beautiful water lily and you are floating on a warm pond. Picture yourself opening up and relaxing, and opening up and relaxing. Imagine your body is drinking in all the energy from the sun and the water, and that this energy will enable you to begin a process of self-love and self-respect which is so strong and complete, you will always be able to point yourself in the right direction without ugly reminders of the past.

That's right, you will now have all the courage and energy necessary to move toward your own highest good simply because of the feeling of self-love emanating from your heart.

You know everything that is and has been happening is actually part of a process enabling you to do what you were meant to do all along. All that has been occurring around you has occurred to free you, so you may go forth into the world and find and create all you are meant to find and create.

As you allow yourself to become fully aware of this, you will be able to forgive all that has occurred. Inside this forgiveness, you will find even more love and freedom.

You know the most important lessons we learn in life are seldom easy to grasp at first, but, as we gain the understanding, it is ours to keep forever.

On this journey today you have learned great lessons, the first one being that your mind wants you to move into a different realm, that it is time for you to create a future for yourself in which you may create your ultimate good.

The second thing you have learned is you must do what is in your best interest, and by doing so, you will be acting in the best interest of everyone concerned.

The third thing you have learned is that you have the capacity to forgive the past and to fully enjoy the future.

Perhaps you have learned more lessons, lessons which were not verbally spoken, lessons which were only heard by your heart and soul. All these lessons will become increasingly apparent in your mind and you will carry them into all the decisions you make today and always. Very good.

Now, Veronica, I'd like you to concentrate on the areas of your body requiring physical healing. I'd like you to focus on these areas and imagine a beautiful, color-filled wave of energy is moving through these areas and returning them to a perfect, healthy state of being. That's right. All the chemical levels, blood sugar, blood pressure, metabolism, veins, vessels, cells, fibers, endocrine glands, and every other functioning feature of your body is coming into perfect harmony and balance. Your body is a marvelous self-healing mechanism and it is now actively creating its own wellness.

Now, you may focus on your heart and soul and allow a color-filled healing energy to move through them. Your own higher self is now speaking healing words which will enable you to feel joy and happiness when the time is right. Your higher self will continually comfort you and remind you that all that is occurring is leading you toward enlightenment.

As you allow your higher self to comfort you, you may allow your heart to sing its song of freedom:

- I am freeing myself from past religious programming and any vows I have taken, which are contradictory to my highest good.

- I am releasing myself from any tendency to automatically follow in the footsteps of my mother and grandmother.

- I behave in a way I know is morally correct and appropriate to my life and times.

- I think clearly and act in my own best interest always.

- By acting in my own best interest, I am automatically acting in the best interest of all those around me.

- Courage and love continually grow inside me.

You may again picture yourself floating like a lily on the surface of a pond. Feel yourself drawing through your soul the light and beauty of the entire universe. Soon the clouds which have been blocking your sun will dissipate and disappear, enabling you to feel the sunshine and see the beauty that the universe sends down to nourish and sustain you. Inside this knowledge and beauty, you will rise up and become all you are meant to be.

Feel yourself becoming energized and clear as I now count from one to five."

I recited the arousal count, and in a moment's time, Veronica was alert and clear.

"How are you doing?"

"I'm fine."

"Do you remember what you said?"

"Yes, I'm sure I do."

"What do you remember?"

"I remember saying my mind was showing me the betrayal over and over again so I would not weaken and run back to Steve."

"That is not exactly what you said, but it does represent the most important part of what you said. Do you remember me asking your mind to let you be free of these pictures and telling it you would act in your best interest without those reminders?"

"Yes. Thank you. I don't think I'll have those dreams anymore. I believe you were right–part of me created them."

"What are you going to do now?"

"I'm going to have to start telling everyone the truth. I can't hide the fact I'm leaving town."

"You're leaving?"

"Yes, I want to go back to LA. I know how to survive there. That will be the best place to start over again. I have friends there and my family will not be far away. I can go out west and recreate myself. So, I'm going to get on my horse and ride into the sunset."

"That sounds exciting. Part of me envies you. I know you can make it on your own–you already are."

Veronica stood up and hugged me. "I think it will take me a couple of weeks to pack-up and get out of here. Should I come see you again?"

"Why don't you see how you feel? You now have the two tapes we made. I think you should keep listening to the tapes, one each day, until you leave. It will help you to stay clear as to what you should do. If you feel like you want another session, call me. I do want you to call me to say good-bye, even if you don't need a session. I'm going to miss you."

TWO WEEKS LATER

Veronica stopped by my office.

"Julie, do you have a minute?"

"Sure. How are you?"

"I'm fine. I wanted to say good-bye and to thank you. I am leaving in a couple of days."

"How have you been holding up?"

"Well, Steve and I have had our screaming matches. He has been trying to get me to go back to him but I haven't budged."

"Did the nightmares stop?"

"Yes, as well as the flashes. I feel very unsettled, but I think under the circumstances, it's normal."

"Of course it is."

"I want you to know the tapes have really helped me. I'm crying less and less, and the future continues to look brighter. I'm scheduled to drive away from here Friday. I keep praying I will have the courage to do it."

"I know you will do the right thing, Veronica."

"I'm glad I started telling my clients the truth about my getting divorced."

"Why, what happened?"

"As I mentioned to you, I was afraid they would judge me for it, but actually, instead of it damaging my reputation, it seems to have done just the opposite."

"How so?"

"My clients have all been coming in for one last appointment and sending me new clients to help before I leave. It's like I'm having a giant going out of business sale. My business has almost tripled since the word of my leaving town got out."

"That is a great testimonial as to how loved you are."

"Yes, it has made me feel loved and appreciated. Everyone has said they admire my ability to do what is right for myself. It really has helped to hear that, but it still all feels so strange. I gave up my home, my husband, my dogs, my friends, my in-laws, and my practice. I feel like I've lost everything but my self-respect."

"That's not true, Veronica."

"It's not?"

"No, you also still have your talent and, with those two things going for you, you will have it all."

"Thanks for saying that. I need to remember that. I'll drop you a line when I find a place to live."

"God bless."

ONE MONTH LATER

Veronica called me from California.

"Julie, I have to tell you what happened the day I left."

"What?"

"I reached a turning point in the road when I was leaving town. I came to a point in the road where I could either continue driving or turn back and go home and say good-bye to Steve and my dogs one last time. I pulled the car off the road and I sat there for the longest time, trying to figure out what to do. I knew if I went back to the house, I might never leave, and I knew it would be easy for me to use my dogs as an excuse to go back."

"What happened?"

"I heard your voice in my head."

"My voice?"

"Yes."

"One of the tapes you made said, one day I would look up into the sky and see a sign which would tell me it was time to finish burying *THE BOOK OF SADNESS*. So, when I didn't know whether I should keep going or turn back, I looked up into the sky to find the sign."

"What did you see?"

"Absolutely nothing."

"Nothing?"

"I looked up and there wasn't a single cloud in the sky. I saw nothing. But then I heard a different voice, it was like my own inner-voice was speaking and it said, 'Look harder, the answer is there.'"

"So, what then?"

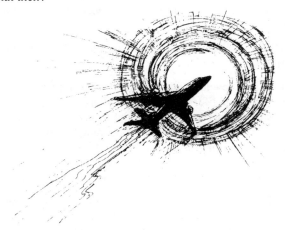

"I stuck my head out of the car window and saw, off in the distance, the white stream a jet leaves behind as it soars away. It was pointing out of town, so I put my foot on the gas pedal and hit the road. I never looked back. Two days later, I was here in LA."

"I'm glad you made it."

Glossary

Abreaction - an emotionally charged physiological response to suggestions made to the subconscious.

Affirmation - statements made to one's self to confirm a belief.

Agoraphobia - a condition in which its sufferers fear going out in public and may be particularly sensitive to being outside in crowds.

Anchor - 1. a factor (which may be a thought, action, memory, sight, sound, or touch) which creates certain feelings and chemical reactions in a person's body. 2. an object which holds another object in place (most often by weighing the object down).

Arousal - the procedure enacted to return an individual from the hypnotized state into normal awareness.

Autism - a life-long developmental disability that typically appears during the first three years of life. The results of a neurological disorder that affects functioning of the brain, some of the behavioral symptoms of autism include: 1. disturbances in the rate of appearance of physical, social, and language skills, 2. abnormal responses to sensations, 3. speech and language are absent or delayed, while specific thinking capabilities may be present, and 4. abnormal ways of relating to people, objects, and events.

Chakras - invisible vortexes of energy in the body which respond to color and musical tones. There are seven major chakras in the human body, each having their own characteristics and functions, and each having a relationship to one of the endocrine system glands as well as one of the colors of the rainbow.

Clearing procedure - a procedure to protect one's own energy supply and to prevent the unhealthful/unhelpful exchange of energy.

Color therapy - the use of color to affect wellness. In hypnotherapy suggestions of color may be utilized to anchor individuals to certain emotions or to create a healing dynamic.

Conscious (mind) - is the part of the mind which keeps the individual in touch with the here and now. The conscious mind possesses a critical factor which weighs out and judges information. The conscious mind is dominant when a person is fully awake and in touch with present day reality.

Creative visualization - the process of visualizing an imaginary scene to serve as a catalyst toward manifesting a desired end result.

Cue - a factor or event which puts a post-hypnotic suggestion into affect or evokes an anchor.

Deepening procedure - a procedure designed to increase the depth of the hypnotic state.

Dissociation - a procedure utilized in hypnotherapy to affect and/or to separate emotional and physical responses to certain stimuli, real, imagined, or recalled. Dissociation is frequently used in regression therapy and to produce hypnoanaesthesia.

Depression - (mental) characterized by an alteration in mood. Depressed persons may present with the following symptoms: a loss of interest in normally enjoyable activities such as food, sex, work, friends, hobbies, or entertainment. Other characteristics of a depressed state may include: decreased sex drive, loss of energy, fatigue, feelings of worthlessness, self-reproach, excessive inappropriate guilt, inability to concentrate and/or diminished focus, recurrent thoughts of death, suicide ideation or attempted. Depression may be caused episodically by grief, or sudden change of life status, or may be organic in nature.

Guided imagery - is the process of one person suggesting to another an imagined scene and outcome.

Hepatitis - an inflammation of the liver.

Higher self - the essence of an individual's highest knowing and deepest beliefs which may present as a separate side of the individual when called upon to do so through hypnosis or related processes.

Hypnosis - a naturally occurring state of altered consciousness (awareness) in which a person is capable of internalizing thought processes for the purpose of affecting profound psychological, physical, and spiritual change. Generally, a hypnotized person has greater awareness of sensations and surroundings, but approximately ten percent of hypnotic subjects go so deeply into hypnosis that they have no conscious recall of the session.

Hypnotherapist - an individual trained and skilled in the use of hypnosis for the purpose of assisting others in creating desired healthy and productive state changes inside their minds, bodies, and lives.

Hypnotic suggestion - suggestions formulated and presented to the subconscious mind for the purpose of creating a state change.

Hypnotist - a person who purposefully induces the state of hypnosis in another.

Ideomotor response - the involuntary capacity of the body to respond to thoughts, feelings, and ideas.

Imbedded commands - secondary commands which are lodged inside of other commands to create two or more reactions simultaneously.

Induction - the procedure enacted to place an individual into the hypnotic state.

Meditation - a state of deep relaxation and mental openness.

Neurolinguistic programming - the study of mind, learning channels, and communication, and the practice of using these components to create wellness and to improve an individual's performance.

NLP - *see neurolinguistic programming.*

Past life regression - the use of hypnosis to enable individuals to mentally recall former existences.

PDR - Physician's Desk Reference (medication guide).

Post-traumatic stress syndrome - a condition caused by emotional or psychological shock which often produces a disordering of feelings, reactions, and behaviors.

Predisposing suggestions - suggestions designed to prepare the subject's mind to accept change.

Progressive relaxation - the act of progressively relaxing the body through thought or suggestion.

Reframing - the act of changing the state/feeling/association of an occurrence from the past via hypnosis.

Regression hypnosis - the use of hypnosis to enable individuals to recall details from the past.

Reincarnation - the belief that individual soul's are repeatedly reborn until they achieve their own human perfection.

Remote - a person who goes into the hypnotic state as a surrogate for another.

Self-hypnosis - is the process of actively hypnotizing one's self.

Subconscious (mind) - the subconscious is the part of the mind which regulates physiological functioning, stores memory, utilizes the imagination, and solves problems. The subconscious is dominant in the following conditions: when a person is sleeping, hypnotized, daydreaming, fantasizing, and/or using imagination or memory.

Suicide - the act of taking one's own life voluntarily.

Trichotillomania - the unnatural impulse to pull out one's own hair.

The Hypnotherapy Training Company's Basic Hypnotherapy Certification Seminar

is open to anyone who wishes to harness the power of his or her own mind for helpful purposes and aspires to help others to do so.

Why Should *You* Attend This Seminar?

The best reason for your attending this program is because you will learn skills of persuasion, self-control, focus, and relaxation that will aid and assist you and those around you for the rest of your life. This program will instantly have a permanent positive effect on how you perceive things and how you do things. You will learn how you can focus your concentration in a positive way that will have a direct impact on your health, happiness, and success in all your endeavors. Upon successful completion of this seminar and the take-home portion of the program, you will be qualified to obtain certification as a hypnotherapist through the American Board of Hypnotherapy.

WHAT YOU WILL LEARN & EXPERIENCE

History of Hypnosis
How Hypnosis Works
Who Can Be Hypnotized
Effective Hypnosis
How to Hypnotize Yourself
Clinical Hypnotherapy
Suggestibility Testing
Anchoring Techniques
Depth Testing
Regression and Progression
How to Recognize Hypnosis

Practical Demonstrations
Hands-On Training
Supervised Student Practice
Sports Hypnosis
Creative Arts Enhancement
Smoking Cessation
Weight Loss
Ethical Hypnosis Practice
Dangers of Hypnosis
Progressive Relaxation
And Much More

Cost for this weekend program is only $445.00 including textbooks. For more information telephone (508) 251-1737 or complete and return form on the last page of this book.

Other Products by Julie Griffin

Recipes for Wellness is a 190–page, thought-provoking collection of 21 hypnotherapy scripts on a wide variety of topics. *Recipes for Wellness* represents the best of Griffin's creative, clinical and spiritual selves. Topics include: weight loss, smoking/alcohol/drug cessation, relaxation & sound sleep, health, creativity, personal power, love & prosperity, happiness, creative writing, enlightenment, golf, memory & learning, birth, death, hypnosis for parents and children, psychic awareness, spirit awareness, past life regression and many more!

Now Available   ISBN 1–57691–000–8   **Price $34.95**

Self-Hypnosis Double-Sided Audio Cassettes

☐ Drawing Love and Prosperity into Your Life/The Happiness Tape

☐ The Optimum Health Tape/Stress Reduction, Relaxation & Sound Sleep

☐ Enhanced Personal Power and Creativity/Enlightenment & Highest Purpose

☐ The Weight Loss Kit

☐ The Stop Smoking Kit

☐ Sexual Enrichment for Men & Women

☐ **Please send me the audio cassettes marked.** I enclosed $19.95 plus $1.50 shipping and handling per double-sided cassette.

☐ **Yes, I want to purchase a copy of *Facilitating Wellness* for a friend.** I enclose $11.95 plus $3.00 shipping and handling.

☐ **I want to purchase a copy of Julie Griffin's scriptbook *Recipes for Wellness*. I enclose $34.95 plus $3.00 shipping and handling.**

☐ **Please send me Julie Griffin's free audio cassette and book catalogue.**

☐ **Please send me free information about *The Hypnotherapy Training Company's* basic and advanced hypnotherapy training programs.**

Name: —————————————— **Tel: (Day)** ——————

Address: ———————————— **(Eve)** ——————

————————————————————————————————————

Checks, Visa, and Mastercard Accepted. MA residents add 5% sales tax.

Card Number: ———————————— **Exp:** ——————

Signature: ————————————————————————

Call Julie Griffin at (508) 251-1737   **TWT Publishing**
or mail this form to: **P. O. Box 2038**
                                                  North Chelmsford, MA 01863